So Your Child Has Diabetes

*A No-nonsense Guide
to Help Your Child Lead
a Normal, Active Life*

Bonnie Estridge and Jo Davies

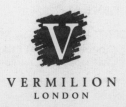

VERMILION
LONDON

Acknowledgements

The authors would like to say a special thankyou to Dr Martin Press MRCP, Hon Senior Lecturer In Medicine at the Charing Cross and Westminster Medical School, for his invaluable help in writing Chapters Eleven and Thirteen.

We would also like to thank the following people for their help, support and encouragement: Anne Corrie (Chief Dietitian at Charing Cross Hospital), the diabetes nurses on the Roehampton Diploma Course, Vanessa Hilton who typed the manuscript, Nick Hilton, Chris Butler, Chris and Hannah Holland, Gloria Ferris, Charlotte Steele, Amanda Cranston, Annaliese Tomkins, Bob Meek, members of the Wimbledon Parent/Family Group and everyone else who helped by contributing their experiences.

FOR SUZY AND CLAIRE

Published in Great Britain by Vermilion
an imprint of the Random Century Group
Random Century House
20 Vauxhall Bridge Road, London SW1V 2SA

Reprinted 1994

A catalogue record for this book is available from the British Library.

ISBN 0 09 177074 2

Typeset in 10/14pt Palatino by M.A.X.
Printed and bound in Great Britain by
Mackays of Chatham PLC, Chatham, Kent

Contents

Preface

There are few things in medicine harder than telling a parent that their child has a serious illness: but it must be even worse for the parent hearing the news. In the case of diabetes it is often made harder still by the fact that it is relatively common, so that most people know someone who has it, and as often as not, there are partial truths and misconceptions which serve only to increase the parents' apprehension.

In the past decade it has finally been realised that in diabetes cases education is of paramount importance. It is important for the child, so that he grows up understanding his condition, and it is equally vital for his parents, not only so that they have the necessary knowledge to cope with their child's diabetes but also so that in due course they can answer their child's questions and help him adjust to his disease. Fortunately, a new health professional, the Diabetes Specialist Nurse, has been created, who has largely taken over the role of educator, a role which in general we doctors had singularly failed to fill.

In this book, Bonnie Estridge, who has a daughter with diabetes and has gone through the traumas of coming to terms with all that the disease entails, has joined forces with Jo Davies, Diabetes Specialist Nurse at Charing Cross Hospital, to produce a guide for the parent of a child with diabetes. It not only provides a veritable encyclopedia of all you need to know about diabetes, but also goes in to the emotional and social aspects of the disease. And although it includes a lot of technical information, it is above all extremely practical.

This book fills a major gap in the market. Although mainly directed at parents of children up to twelve years old, it will be of immense value to parents of children of any age with diabetes, and I am flattered to have been asked to contribute two chapters. Many of the problems which we encounter in adults with diabetes are due to poor education in childhood: the first few days and weeks of the disease often shape their attitudes for the rest of their lives. This book offers guidance which will, in due course, result in fewer problems for people with diabetes not only in childhood but throughout the rest of their lives.

Martin Press
Hon Senior Lecturer in Medicine
Charing Cross & Westminster Medical School

Introduction

Whether your child has been newly diagnosed or has had diabetes for some time you will know that it's for life. At first you may feel bewildered, depressed and simply bogged down by the paraphernalia of injections, blood testing and diet. It's natural to feel shocked – devastated is a word used frequently by parents of newly diagnosed children – or even guilty for something you imagine you have done wrong in the upbringing of your child.

The aim of this book is to go into as many areas of a child's lifestyle as possible and help you, as parents, fit diabetes into family living.

Diabetes will never go away but it certainly need not take over your life. The key to smooth diabetes management is normality. Ideally, your child should lead a completely normal life with the chores of insulin injections and blood tests fitting routinely in with everyday living.

A relaxed, responsible diabetic child needs a relaxed, responsible parent. Children with diabetes need parents who don't lose sleep over how many chips their offspring has eaten at tea. They do not need mum appearing at a birthday party wielding a syringe or waking them up in the dead of night for unnecessary blood tests. They need a routine they can understand and sometimes bend to suit their lifestyle. With today's array of high-tech blood testing equipment you will be able to monitor your child's sugar levels and try to keep them as near normal as is possible. But it's almost impossible to achieve perfection. Blood sugar readings are not exam results and you should aim for the best control as is possible under the prevailing circumstances; diabetes is an erratic condition.

By giving the best possible start to controlling diabetes it is widely believed that future health risks are minimised. Encouraging your child to be independent and relaxed will pay dividends – confidence can flourish as she grows up determined not to let diabetes interfere with living life to the full.

The British Diabetic Association (BDA) is a huge organisation that will provide invaluable links with other parents who have a child with diabetes and gives information on all the new developments that are going on around the world. As a member of the BDA you will never feel cut off and alone.

You will be finding out – to your relief – that modern thinking about the value of food has revolutionised the diabetic diet. In fact, there are a lot of negative things you may have thought applied to diabetics that simply do not. We hope that this book will help take the hassle out of day-to-day living with diabetes for your child and, indeed, the whole family. We hope to cover situations that beg questions you may feel reluctant to ask busy medical staff; things you feel they may consider trivial yet loom large in your family's needs. The idea of this book is to take away the strain and help you cope with what is becoming an increasingly common condition. We have gathered together many comments from other parents who have diabetic children and these are interwoven through the chapters to help you learn from their experiences.

Both authors have close female relatives who are diabetic, but for reasons of convenience in writing this book we refer to the child as 'he', or 'she' in alternate chapters.

Chapter 1

Understanding Diabetes

'I couldn't believe how much Harry was drinking . . .'

'My five year old daughter was constantly on the toilet . . .'

'Emily lost so much weight we feared she had cancer . . .'

*'All we knew was that diabetes had something to
do with sugar . . .'*

What is Diabetes?

Diabetes is a serious condition which results if the pancreas, a gland close to the stomach and the liver, fails to work properly. Normally, the pancreas makes a hormone called insulin which is vital for processing glucose (sugar) in the body. Sometimes, a person's pancreas fails to produce any, or enough, insulin, and glucose, instead of being burnt by the body to produce energy, remains in the blood, and eventually spills over into the urine. A person with diabetes, if left untreated, will fall ill and eventually die, because their body is not receiving vital energy from glucose to keep it going.

Diabetes as an illness has been recognised for thousands of years yet it is only quite recently that we have been able to treat it successfully. The full name of the condition is *diabetes mellitus*. The Greek translation of this is 'fountain of honey' which is an apt description for the sickly sweet urine that is passed when there is a high level of sugar (glucose) in the blood.

For centuries, apart from strange brews and potions given to try and

LOCATION OF PANCREAS

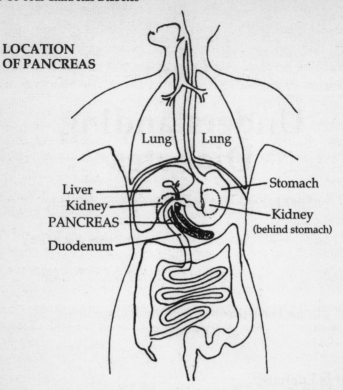

Lung Lung

Liver
Kidney
PANCREAS
Duodenum

Stomach
Kidney
(behind stomach)

cure the disease – with no success – a near starvation diet was the only short-term alternative. Sufferers eventually died from malnutrition. During the late 19th century doctors discovered that the removal of a dog's pancreas led to symptoms of diabetes and this provided the first clue to the problem. However, it was not then known which ingredient found in the pancreas was missing in people who had diabetes.

In 1921 two scientists, Frederick Banting and Charles Best, working through their summer holidays at the University of Toronto discovered the importance of insulin. The pancreas releases essential digestive juices which enable food to be absorbed into the body. However, of more importance is the fact that the pancreas also produces various hormones which flow directly into the bloodstream, as Banting and Best found. Insulin is the most crucial of these hormones because it helps convert sugar (from the food we eat) to energy and store it in cells around the body. It was this lack of insulin that led to diabetes and, before this discovery, to certain death.

A fourteen year old boy who lay dying of the disease in the Toronto General Hospital was the first human to be treated with insulin. The boy made a remarkable recovery and insulin replacement was hailed as a miracle cure which, to all intents and purposes, it still is.

Through lack of insulin, the body of a diabetic cannot make normal use of sugar and the level of sugar in the blood rises way beyond the normal limit. This is known as hyperglycaemia. Soon, the kidneys cannot cope with this 'overloading', sugar is discharged into the urine creating the 'fountain of honey'. If you ever smelled (or even tasted) your child's urine before diagnosis you would have found it pungently sweet. In the end, survival is impossible without the store of sugar to provide energy because the body will 'feed from itself' by breaking down fat and protein in order to obtain energy. At this advanced stage serious illness is inevitable and the array of unpleasant symptoms associated with diabetes really show themselves.

Symptoms of Diabetes in Your Child

Several parents have told us during our research for this book that they could pin-point the exact time their child showed the first signs of diabetes, as its onset can be very sudden indeed. However, the diabetes may have been brewing for months – even years, but very early symptoms can be masked by other factors (for example drinking a lot in very hot weather).

One mother reported: 'It was 2 pm on the Sunday after Christmas and we had stopped at a petrol station en route to my husband's parents. My daughter asked for some chocolate and then threw a complete tantrum because they didn't have the bar she wanted. She was nearly seven and past this two-year-old kind of behaviour. It was completely out of character as she threw herself around the garage forecourt screaming and crying. Once she had calmed down and we had arrived at her grandparents she spent the next four hours drinking constantly, and I reprimanded her for being rude as she kept going to the kitchen and helping herself to drinks.

The drinking continued when we got home and she called several times in the night. My husband had a routine medical the next day so I asked him to take her urine sample for testing. I had heard about this crazed drinking in diabetes but I didn't really expect this to be the outcome.'

Another mother actually found her young son, aged five, sucking the overflow pipe from the washing machine after she had banned him from a seemingly endless drinking spree. 'There had to be something wrong. Once I'd put a stop to that he went to the cat's bowl and began licking it like an animal. I cannot describe how guilty I felt when he was diagnosed as having diabetes.'

These parents may not have noticed that their children were also passing large amounts of urine, or they may have thought that this was a result of all the drinking. In fact, it's the frequent toilet trips that give rise to the burning thirst. There is so much excess sugar in the blood that water has to be taken from other cells in the body to dilute it and is then passed out from the kidneys. This is dehydrating and leads to the need to drink and replace lost fluids. A number of parents have missed these early signals due to the weather being hot and everyone in general feeling thirsty. Bed-wetting is another common symptom arising from the frequent need to pass water. Some parents realised something was badly amiss, but again, and especially with young children, this could have been put down to all the drinking, or other problems at school or home.

Unfortunately some parents were told by their GPs, rather bluntly, that there was no need to test the child as many children tended to ask for drinks through habit and the bed-wetting could be 'just a stage they are going through'.

Another symptom of diabetes is itching around the genitals. This happens because of all the sugar in the urine and often develops into thrush. Again, this may have been ignored or treated as a common childhood complaint. Your child may have complained about blurred vision; this happens when sugar fills the lens of the eye and vision becomes distorted. This does go back to normal after treatment has started although it may take some weeks.

As we explained earlier, one of the jobs of insulin is to change sugar into energy. When your child is not making enough insulin to manage this, her body has to make energy from other sources. So, fat and protein are broken down to compensate. This causes the child to lose weight and most parents become worried when a child loses weight very quickly despite an increase in appetite. Some children only lose a few pounds or kilos, while others can lose as much as two stone [12.7 kilos].

You may have noticed a strange smell on your child's breath – rather like pear drops or nail-polish remover. This is due to *ketones* in the blood. Ketones are harmful chemicals which appear when body fat is being broken down and the smell is due to a substance called acetone (see page 61).

This breakdown of fat and protein, or 'fat meltdown', also causes tiredness and a feeling of weakness. You may have noticed your child falling asleep at odd times. Tiredness inevitably leads to irritability and many parents told us of poor performance at school which was being put down to the usual teachers' complaint: 'lack of concentration'.

'George had been doing so well in his first year at primary school that we were quite shocked when his third end of term report said his reading had gone downhill and he appeared to be sleeping during many of his lessons,' one mother told us. 'Within a month George was taking insulin and he had changed completely. The teachers could not believe it and apologised, saying how guilty they felt.'

Once treated with insulin there is a very fast improvement in the child and all these symptoms disappear. You may even think that there has been some ghastly mistake and the diabetes has now gone away. Unfortunately it hasn't and it won't. But at least your child will have been restored to her former healthy self.

How ill your child actually becomes before diabetes is diagnosed rather depends on how early the symptoms are spotted. Many parents blame themselves for not having noticed warning signs. One mother genuinely believed her twelve year old daughter was a hypochondriac, trying to compete with her asthmatic brother, and secretly wanting to lose weight. The feeling of relief when a child responds quickly to treatment may not wipe out feelings of guilt and sometimes anger – at a GP who refused to take the initial problem seriously. However, although diabetes is becoming far more common, as we shall see later in this chapter, it is not found on a scale like chickenpox or mumps. And it is not an illness that immediately springs to mind unless someone has close contact with another diabetic. If it took considerable time to diagnose your child, please don't blame yourself; take comfort in the fact that your child has been treated successfully and can now enjoy good health.

It is upsetting to hear that a small number of GPs were reluctant to perform a simple urine test and diagnosis was missed until a child became really ill. It is up to those who have a knowledge of diabetes to urge others, who may have been rebuffed by a busy or unsympathetic GP, either to insist on a urine test if they have reason to be concerned, or to go elsewhere for a second opinion.

Why My Child?

No one really knows what causes diabetes. You will, however, be amazed at how common this condition is becoming. Everyone, it seems, knows someone who is diabetic. And that, in an odd way, may give you comfort.

There are over 600,000 people in the UK alone registered as diabetics, but they are not all dependent on insulin. A child who produces little or no insulin will have to rely on treatment for the rest of his or her life. This Type 1, or insulin-dependent diabetes, usually develops between birth and the age of forty. Older people who have Type 2 or non-insulin-dependent diabetes still produce some insulin and are able to control their blood sugars by a careful diet, tablets, or a combination of both. Worldwide, there are an estimated thirty million people with diabetes and around twenty-five per cent of these are insulin dependent. In the last twenty years the incidence rate of insulin-dependent diabetes in children under fifteen living in the UK has doubled and three thousand new cases are now being diagnosed annually.

The big question – and one which is now of great public health concern – is why? Many people share a belief that diabetes is an inherited disorder and it would be true to say that certain families carry a strong tendency to develop the disease. But in many new cases parents are unable to trace one relative with diabetes on either side of the family. It seems likely, though, that many people carry a gene or susceptibility towards diabetes and if something occurs to trigger it, the full-blown illness will then develop. It has been suggested that diabetes can develop as a result of a shock such as an accident or even a major upheaval such as a child starting a new school. Although a shock will not actually cause diabetes, the emotional stress may bring on an increase in blood sugar and may trigger the diabetes which the child was already developing. Scientists are constantly trying to find out what precipitates diabetes. It is possible that the cause may be environmental but actually uncovering a cause does seem to be a long way off.

Diabetes often appears to start in young people after a viral illness or infection such as a cold and it is widely suspected that some kind of virus (as yet unidentified) is the cause. However, there is *no* actual diabetes virus and it is impossible to 'catch' diabetes from someone else. Only in a person who carries the tendency in their genes and then catches the 'trigger' virus will diabetes occur. The chances of your child passing on diabetes to future children are one in twenty for a man and one in a hundred for a woman. If both parents are diabetic the chances are higher, yet many children of diabetic parents never develop the disease.

We were told about two pairs of identical twins where one twin has become diabetic and the other has not. Parents have naturally found this especially hard to deal with.

Hospitals and clinics report a rise in cases at certain times of the year, most notably during the late winter months. This seems to back up the virus/trigger theory as more colds and infections are around in late winter. It has also been noted that the peak time for children of either sex to develop diabetes occurs during puberty.

Please rest assured that there is absolutely nothing you or anyone else could have done to prevent your child developing diabetes. It is common for parents to feel that they made mistakes over their child's diet. Perhaps you are worried that she ate too many sweets or junk foods: this has been totally ruled out by doctors and scientists. There is simply nothing you could have done to stop diabetes happening and now your goal must be to make life for your child relaxed and normal.

Your Child Really *Can* Live a Normal Life

Can your child lead a normal life with a strict daily routine of injections and diet? You may worry that she will become a semi-invalid, forever being off school 'sick', passing out all over the place and being unable to join in sport or normal activities that other children take for granted. This is most definitely not the case and as you read through this book you will see that there is no reason to change any part of your child's lifestyle. Apart from the mechanics of insulin treatment (which, please believe it, will become second nature and take very little time indeed) you can let life go on as usual.

Extra planning will no doubt be needed but you will become an expert at foreseeing snags along the way and thus be forearmed. There is no trip that cannot be taken and no circumstances that cannot be overcome as long as you are well organised .

As for days off school, statistics show that children with diabetes frequently have a better record of attendance than their non-diabetic counterparts and often fare better than average in exams. Perhaps they feel the need to prove that they are just as normal as everyone else! Once insulin treatment has started and the dose is found to be right you will notice how healthy your child looks and many parents have told us that their diabetic offspring shake off colds and other childhood illnesses far quicker than siblings. It's true that a bad bout of illness can be hard to control with blood sugars needing extra attention (see Chapter Nine) but the majority of children with diabetes are robust, healthy and tough. You may also find that a previously introverted child gains new confidence from being that little bit 'special'. Despite the fact that their lifestyle may be completely normal they will always feel different from the crowd and this can have a very positive effect.

A number of parents have told us of a new extrovert in the family: a child who has something that is completely to do with her and a knowledge of her own body that not many adults have. Your child will certainly feel 'different' in a negative way if you give her those signals. If you are forever using diabetes as an excuse not to let her do anything or go anywhere she will soon learn to hate it. Even if the injection/mealtime routine doesn't seem to fit into the outing she wants to go on, don't say no – give it some thought. There are ways round almost every situation as you will see later in this book.

Children do not like to appear outwardly different and unless diabetes is treated as an obstacle they will soon realise that nobody can actually see anything odd about them. They may choose to let friends watch blood tests and injections and often enjoy the attention and interest given. They become toughened to whimpers of 'I could never do injections' or 'You are so brave . . . I'd hate that' and may show a certain amount of ambivalence towards less courageous friends. Think positively – diabetes can be character-building.

There will also be children who bitterly resent their diabetes and grow up to feel that they are in some way flawed or less than perfect. But who gave them that idea in the first place?

It's normal that your child may feel sad at times and show strong feelings of anger which may be directed towards herself, you or the world in general. Anger is a very physical emotion and perhaps you should encourage your child to put it to good use instead of letting it generate endless rows at home. Sport is a great way of letting off steam. Let the child participate in as many activities as possible to use up excess energy. A punchbag to take swipes at is a harmless recipient of knock-out blows – for either sex.

Anger can also be used creatively to express emotions in writing, drawing or painting. It can also be used musically: it is well known from his music how Beethoven felt about being deaf.

Encourage your child to talk openly and share her feelings with others. Don't let her feel that diabetes is a taboo subject or anything to be ashamed of. She may grow to dislike the total dependence on insulin yet you can help her realise that all of us are dependent on things or people right through our lives.

There are certain perks in the life of the child with diabetes too: the chocolate bar (banned to other pupils) before PE at school, the mid-morning snack . . . not many children would consider this a disadvantage.

When these children grow up there is no reason at all why they should not get married and have healthy children of their own. Girls will obviously need a good understanding of the importance of blood sugar control before and during pregnancy but they will, of course, be carefully monitored throughout. Fertility in either sex is no different from that in a non-diabetic so an understanding of contraception is as vital for diabetics as it is for everyone else.

A career in the forces, flying a plane or scuba-diving may be 'out' for the diabetic but there is very little else that is insurmountable. Many top sports personalities, actors and professionals are diabetic. Suffice to say that the more low-key approach you take with your child in the beginning, the easier diabetes will fit into her life. Children are resilient and flexible. They can adapt to strange circumstances far quicker and with less anxiety than adults can. Even if you experience problems at the beginning, careful handling should resolve them and your child will, in all probability, accept diabetes into the daily routine and get on with life.

Chapter 2

The First Few Days

'I felt as if my whole world had collapsed . . .'

'We were sure the doctors had made a mistake . . .'

'I was devastated – so shocked I could hardly think straight . . .'

'Frightened! I thought I was going to lose her.'

Emotional Reactions

These are just some of the feelings experienced by parents of newly diagnosed diabetic children. To be told your child has diabetes will come as a shock even if you had anticipated the diagnosis and thought you had prepared yourself. Or you may not even have ever heard of diabetes, or thought it was something only old people developed.

Many parents experience a sense of loss and feel they no longer have a perfect child. You may feel angry: 'What have I done? Why me?' You may even feel your child has let you down. Some parents take out their anger on a partner or other children. Some also find themselves venting frustrations on the doctors and nurses caring for the child because there is no cure or nothing easier than injections. 'What about tablets? How about this cell transplant I've heard about?' Some people will grasp at straws, hoping that there might be 'just something'.

Guilt is one of the strongest emotions parents feel. Some blame themselves, without reason, for 'passing on' diabetes. You may find yourself looking round for a cause. 'I thought I had let her eat too many sweets,' one mother told us. Another parent thought the severe telling off her son had received the week before had triggered off his diabetes. 'He didn't have diabetes before then.' But this is not so. She just did not know about his condition at the time. Know that *nothing* you have said or done has caused your child's diabetes.

We also asked parents who either had diabetes themselves or who had a family history of insulin-dependent diabetes how they felt. Feelings were mixed. One family said they cannot imagine how they would have coped had the father of their child not had diabetes. They felt they had an advantage as they already knew about diabetes and their son had often watched his father give injections and do blood tests. Other parents felt guilty because they had 'passed on' a lifelong condition. However, it must be remembered that new technology is making life easier for people with diabetes all the time. Even something as simple as plastic syringes has revolutionised their lives. Some of you reading this book will remember having to boil glass syringes to sterilise them, then keep them in industrial spirit. Sounds archaic doesn't it? Bear in mind a lot has happened in *your* lifetime and a lot more will happen in your child's.

You will be aware that your child will also be going through emotional turmoil. Like you, he will ask 'Why me?' He may also imagine that he has caused his diabetes, perhaps because he was naughty last week or fought with his brother or sister. Children don't always express how they feel so it is important to reassure your child that *he* has not caused the diabetes, even if he never suggests this is the case. Children also have a different concept of illness to adults. Illness to a child is something which may require them to stay at home or in hospital where they have to take medicine or injections to make them better. As far as they are concerned, when they are better the medicine and injections should stop. The problem with diabetes is that the injections carry on. This is even more difficult for the child who has not felt particularly unwell; indeed, he will have great difficulty understanding why he has to have injections at all. On top of all this he is being told when he can and cannot eat certain foods. All this results in his feeling very confused.

You and the medical staff will have to keep explaining the reason for the injections and the sweet restrictions repeatedly. If there are brothers and sisters in the family they will also be upset and possibly frightened, especially if the child is admitted to hospital. They, too, will need an explanation about diabetes and why their brother or sister needs injections and blood tests. Your explanation should prevent any looks or sounds of fear or disdain from siblings which might result in your diabetic child refusing to have his insulin injections.

A simple way of explaining diabetes to a young child might be: 'Something inside Mary's tummy is not working which means too much sugar is in her blood. This could make her ill and the injections are a medicine which helps take the sugar away. Too many sweets stop the medicine working so Mary will not be able to eat them all the time, but she will be able to have some as treats.'

The first few days will probably be bewildering. Many parents have likened diabetes to a 'maze'. You will find yourself worrying about day-to-day living. Thoughts of how, when and why will crowd your head.

'How will we cope with the injections? She has enough problems with school vaccinations.'
'I've never stuck to a diet – how will I manage with this?'
'When will we *do* the injections?'
'It's her birthday next week and I've promised a party.'

Just take one thing at a time. You won't be expected to be an expert in diabetes overnight. If your child is feeling better then there is no need to cancel the party; if you do, your child will immediately feel resentful towards her diabetes. There will be times in the following months, even years, when you may feel sad; particularly on occasions like birthdays or Christmas. These feelings will fade with time. Some parents have likened their child's development of diabetes to bereavement. It does take time to come to terms with it and no-one expects you to accept diabetes calmly right away.

Don't bottle up your emotions or you will cause yourself a great deal of stress. Share your thoughts with your family and friends, doctor or nurse. However, beware of any family or friends who tell you 'horror' stories about complications. If you hear any of these *don't* dwell on them or else *you* will worry yourself sick. Tell your doctor or diabetes nurse. They will be able to explain the facts; (and we will talk about this subject more in Chapter Four). Remember your doctor and nurse are there to help you and your family, so do ask questions. It is often useful and reassuring to talk to another parent who has been through the same emotional turmoil as yourself. Your diabetes nurse or doctor should be able to arrange this for you, as can the British Diabetic Association (BDA), which organises a Parent Network. Many parents described an overwhelming sense of relief when they heard how others were coping. In most cases they were told: 'Don't worry, it will all click and it's not nearly as bad as it seems right now.' The key to coming to terms with and understanding diabetes is communication. This is not just down to you; it is vital for the doctor, nurse and dietitian to communicate with you.

Hospital or Home?

Depending on how ill your child is and the type of diabetes service you have in your area will dictate whether he is admitted to hospital or remains at home.

Some children who are admitted to hospital are severely ill. These children will be very dehydrated. As we explained in Chapter One, the high level of sugar in the blood draws fluid from the surrounding cells to dilute the sugary blood which passes through the kidneys, leading to an increase in the amount of urine passed. This leads to the terrific thirst. The severely ill child will also be very weak and may even be in a coma. He will also have lost a considerable amount of weight, because of ketones in the body. Ketones are formed when the body breaks down fat to make energy, because there is not enough insulin to break down sugar to make energy. It is important to remember that ketones are dangerous. They are a poisonous acid and when there is a build-up of ketones due to a severe lack of insulin over a period of time it leads to *ketoacidosis* (sometimes called *ketosis* or *diabetic coma*) which produces the dramatic symptoms of vomiting, nausea, stomach pain, shortness of breath and, unless treated, eventually coma. Parents whose children are admitted to hospital naturally feel intense fear, particularly if their child is semi-conscious. Some children may even be admitted to the intensive care unit but fortunately this is rare.

One mother explained how everything happened in a rush; one minute she was in casualty with her son, the next he was being surrounded by medical staff and whisked off to the ward. 'Nobody explained what they were doing with James, or what they were going to do. It all happened so quickly.'

Another mother described her reaction when she first saw her son on the ward. 'I went behind the curtains and felt absolutely petrified. He was attached to drips and surrounded by gadgetry. I now know that one of the gadgets was only a blood glucose meter – but I wasn't to know that then.'

The drips and gadgets include a bag of fluid to replace the fluid your child lost when he was passing so much urine. There will also be a pump, pumping insulin into your child as he can no longer make his own. The amount will depend on his blood sugar levels. This will be measured by pricking your child's finger hourly to get a sample of blood so that the sugar can be measured at the bedside. Rest assured your child will not be having hourly finger pricks for life! But he and you will have to learn how to do this, as the blood sugar levels will have to be monitored from time to time at home to see if he is getting the right amount of insulin. Doctors will also be taking blood samples which will be sent to the laboratory. This is not a finger prick but usually involves a small needle being inserted into the hand or arm. (Some doctors put on a cream to numb the area first.) These blood tests will tell the doctor how out of balance the body chemicals are, and also allow a double check on the blood sugar. Most importantly, these tests will show the doctor how much progress is being made. Your child's urine will also be tested for ketones. Eventually these will disappear as there

is now insulin available to convert sugar into energy and so he is
no longer breaking down fat. (How insulin works is explained in
Chapter Three). He is now on the road to recovery and you will
soon notice an improvement in his condition.

Fortunately, most children are not severely ill. They will probably
have the symptoms, but may insist they do not feel particularly
unwell. Sometimes it is only when they have started insulin
treatment and feel better that they recognise how tired or thirsty
they were feeling. Mildly affected children might be admitted to
hospital for a number of reasons: for example, there may not be
adequate services in the area to support and help educate the
family at home at that particular time. However, a number of
parents told us their child was admitted at the weekend and
because the diabetes team were not on duty there was no one to
explain about diabetes to them. Some parents, when given the
choice of home or hospital, chose hospital. This gave them a
breather after the traumatic time they had recently gone through. It
also gave them time to talk to their families and begin learning
how to cope with the new situation. Although some families were
relieved that their child was admitted to hospital there were some
who found it very difficult, particularly if there were siblings. One
parent stayed with the newly diagnosed child whilst the other
looked after the other children, and although these parents
received support from the hospital staff they desperately wanted to
be able to discuss fears and thoughts with their partner. Single
parents met with a lot of difficulties, especially those who had
other children. One mother felt guilty that she could not stay with
her child all night in the hospital, as she had others at home.

We were concerned to hear about some of the ways in which
parents were told about their child's diagnosis in hospital. Even if
your family doctor has already told you your child has diabetes, on
admission to hospital this should be explained to you again, not
because your GP was wrong, but, like many parents you want to
be sure a mistake has not been made. You may not quite believe
what you have already been told, or you may not want to believe it
and imagine that the whole thing is happening to someone else! In

one case a parent seemed to wait a 'lifetime' before the diagnosis was confirmed. This obviously causes a lot of anxiety.

Sadly, not all parents were told in a sympathetic and understanding manner. One senior registrar 'mentioned it in passing'. The parents had no idea their child had diabetes until he matter-of-factly started a sentence with: 'So your child has diabetes . . .'. The parents were understandably left reeling. In some cases there seemed to be a lack of team work between the doctor and the diabetes specialist nurse. We heard of one incident where there was a violent disagreement in front of the parent and child. Also, the ward nurses were not always familiar with diabetes. One mother told us: 'The nurses on the ward did not appear to know what Harry could or could not eat and he had a very unhappy first evening.'

Fortunately complaints about hospital staff were in the minority. More often they came in for a lot of praise. 'The doctor was very kind. He took my family into a room and explained in simple language what diabetes meant.' As a family, the *diabetes specialist nurse* is the person who you will probably come into most contact with. Over the first few days you will begin to understand what diabetes in your family's life really means. The diabetes specialist nurse will show you what is involved when giving insulin, performing blood or urine tests and much more besides. There should also be a visit from the dietitian to provide information and advice about the type of food your diabetic child (and your family) should be eating.

However, not all children are admitted to hospital. Those who are not unwell and who live in an area where there are good support services may be treated at home with the consent of the parents. The advantage of starting treatment at home is that life for the child carries on as normal and hopefully diabetes is a low-key rather than a major event. The family will receive advice and support either from the hospital team, or from the GP and health visitor who will visit at home. Once treatment has started, the child will return to school and carry on normal activities. But there can be disadvantages with this system. Firstly, it is difficult for the child to understand why he has to have injections when he does not feel ill. This takes some explaining so let the doctor or nurse help you. Secondly, the parents do not get a break and may feel they are shouldering too much responsibility too soon. Although they make home visits regularly, the doctor or nurse cannot be there twenty-four hours a day. However, there is usually a contact telephone number for any problems or worries. Some parents like this system of care; being 'thrown in at the deep end' teaches them quickly and it is less disruptive for the child and the rest of the family. Some families may not be visited at home, instead they go to see the doctor and diabetes specialist nurse at the hospital on a daily basis. As confidence grows, hospital visits become less frequent, and you can always get in touch with the hospital by phone.

Once your child starts receiving insulin you will notice an improvement – dramatically in some cases. One father commented: 'We knew Thomas was getting better when he started arguing with his brother!' You will feel immense relief when you see your child 'getting back to his old self'. The next few days and weeks may be a trying time, but you will eventually find that you have come out of that 'maze'.

In the beginning you will meet a number of staff involved in your child's care and you may be unsure what is expected of *you*. You will see the doctor frequently in the first few days. Do ask questions. It may help to write them down, then you will not forget what you want to ask. All children with diabetes should be under the care of a hospital whether treatment started at home or in hospital. You will be asked to attend an out-patient clinic after your child leaves hospital (this applies to those starting treatment at home, too). At this clinic you will see:

The Doctor

Whether your child was diagnosed by your GP or the hospital doctor he should have a medical examination, at the time of diagnosis, by a doctor who has experience in looking after children. In hospital this doctor is usually a *paediatrician* (someone who specialises in children's medicine). However, this doctor may be someone who works in the diabetes department (a *diabetologist*) and has knowledge of children's medicine. At home it could be your GP. In many hospitals the paediatrician and the diabetologist run joint clinics so you might see them both when you visit the out-patients' department. At the clinic visits, the doctor will look at a 'diary' showing the blood sugars or urine tests you and your child have done at home and may alter the insulin dose accordingly. In the beginning you may find the insulin dose altered frequently, a little at a time. This is because the doctor (or the diabetes nurse) is trying to find the right dose of insulin to maintain a normal blood glucose level. You will not always see the doctor or nurse because, eventually, given time and confidence, you will be able to work out the change in insulin dose for yourself. How frequently you see the hospital doctor in the beginning will be up to the two of you. However, it is most important your child has at least one annual check-up for the rest of his life.

Between the times you see the doctor you will see:

The Diabetes Specialist Nurse

You may know her as the diabetes care sister/nurse or diabetes liaison sister and you will probably call her by her Christian name. This is the person with whom you will have most contact. She may be a health visitor, a practice nurse or a nurse who only works in the field of diabetes. Whoever she is she must have a sound knowledge of diabetes and be able to communicate well with children and their families.

In the beginning, it will be she who helps you learn about diabetes and the practical aspects of day-to-day living. She understands there is a lot for you and your child to take in and will try not to overload you with information. But there are certain things, such as injections, which you will learn right from the beginning. Your diabetes nurse will give you advice and support. She does not mind being inundated with questions or being a shoulder to cry on (really!). Most diabetes nurses will try and see you on a daily basis in the beginning, especially if your child is at home. She will continue to see you as often as you and she feel is necessary. Make sure you know how to contact your diabetes specialist nurse if you have any problems – she will want you to. Most nurses have a contact number. Don't be afraid to use it – that's what it's for! No, you will not be a nuisance or a bother. As you become more confident in your understanding you will see her less and less. Eventually you and your child will become the experts in diabetes.

You will also come into contact with:

The Dietitian

As with the doctor and the diabetes specialist nurse the dietitian should have good knowledge of the dietary needs for children. Most dietitians are based in hospital although some are community based. You may see the dietitian in the hospital, at your GP's surgery, or she may even visit your home.

She will take a diet history; this means she will ask precisely what your child eats during a day. She will assess if your child is eating the right foods for both growth and diabetes, and explain any modifications you may have to make. The dietitian will try to make as little change as possible; she will be realistic while taking your child's likes and dislikes into account.

A number of visual aids are used in dietary education, which help children (and adults) remember what they are taught. She will probably have plastic models of foods and empty food cartons to show you. Even if your child is too young to understand, he will enjoy playing with some of the food models! If you come across a food you are not sure is suitable, write down the name and ask the dietitian. Diet is one of the biggest problems that parents imagine they will face, but you will soon find out that a 'diabetes diet' is normal healthy eating and usually suitable for all the family. Obviously, if your child has had a previous dietary problem, such as allergies to dairy foods or wheat products, then this will have to be taken into account.

Once again you will be in regular contact at the beginning. It is important your child has regular dietary assessments as his needs will change throughout his life. The subject of diet will be covered in Chapter Six.

So, now you know what the healthcare professionals do, you may be wondering exactly what is expected of you.

The Parents

You have the most difficult job simply because you cannot go home and forget about diabetes. At the moment it is the foremost thing in your mind, but it will not always be like that. Your job is to keep the 'professionals' informed. Let them know if your child has a 'hypo' (see page 45). Keep a record of the tests you do. Inform them of high sugar levels or swings in the blood/urine tests (highs and lows). Let them know how you and your child are getting along with the injections and what problems you are having, if any. Tell them how your child is coping with the finger pricks; these sometimes cause more bother than the injections. What about the diet? Is your child upset because he cannot have as much chocolate as he used to? Let them know of any little problem that bothers you, your child or your family. They are sure to be able to help you work it out. Your medical team will ask you about some of these matters but not all of them communicate effectively, as we have found out! To get out of the 'maze' you sometimes have to ask the way.

Chapter 3

All About Insulin

'The injections just become a rather annoying part of life . . .'

'Insulin injections are now the key to your child's life. However much you hate that idea there is no way out . . .'

'My eight year old will happily inject himself – but only in total silence. He almost meditates! If we're out and it's noisy then I have to inject him – he has to concentrate totally . . .'

The Miracle Treatment

The first person to receive insulin was fourteen year old Leonard Thompson in January 1922. Since then, the discovery of insulin has saved millions of lives. Natural insulin is produced in the pancreas. The actual cells that produce it are the Beta Cells which lie within the Islets of Langerhans, another group of cells in the pancreas. Insulin is a hormone and also a protein-like substance. The reason that it has to be injected is because if it were taken by mouth it would be digested and destroyed before it reached the bloodstream.

You may have heard of older people with diabetes taking tablets and wonder whether this might be an alternative for your child. Unfortunately this would not solve the problem. In older people the tablets used are to stimulate the pancreas to produce *more* insulin (because it is still functioning) and the tablets are drugs, not hormones. However, they are very rarely suitable in the treatment of children. In fact, many children actually find injections easier.

How Insulin Works

Insulin is injected to lower the blood sugar levels which rise after each meal. Regular meals or snacks are needed to prevent the insulin from making the sugar levels drop too low. Looking at how the body acts in a non-diabetic person may make it easier to understand why your child needs regular injections of insulin.

Sugar in the blood comes from the food we eat, in particular from carbohydrates. These can be in the form of sweet foods like cakes, biscuits and chocolate or in the form of starchy foods like bread, potatoes, rice or pasta. After a meal, or even a snack, the sugar from these foods is absorbed into the bloodstream causing a rise in blood sugar. A rise in blood sugar stimulates the beta cells to produce insulin, which is also released into the bloodstream.

Because your child cannot produce insulin, the blood sugar level continues to rise, leading to *hyperglycaemia*. This is the medical term for high blood sugar ('hyper' means high, 'hypo' means low). Insulin also enables sugar to enter the body cells where it is converted into energy. The blood sugar level usually falls back to normal about two hours after food.

Any sugar which is not used to provide energy immediately is stored for later use. It is stored either as fat, or in the liver as glycogen which can be changed back into sugar when extra energy is needed. When there is no insulin to convert sugar into energy your child experiences the symptoms we have previously described and this is why she needs regular injections of insulin to keep her blood sugar levels normal.

Never stop your child's insulin – even if she is ill or vomiting.

What is Normal?

Throughout EEC countries the amount of sugar in the blood is measured in millimoles per litre (mmol/l). Four millimoles (4mmol) is the equivalent of a quarter of a teaspoonful of sugar. You will have a better idea of what this measurement means if you visualise a quarter teaspoonful of sugar in one litre of water. The range of blood sugars found in a non-diabetic person is very narrow. Even after meals it usually stays between 3.5 and 8mmol/l unless strenuous exercise causes it to drop or undue stress due to, say, a car accident causes it to rise. But the kind of blood sugar fluctuations seen in diabetics would never be found in a non-diabetic.

Without insulin in the body, the amount of sugar in the blood can rise to as much as ten times the normal level (even more sometimes) and the function of the insulin injections is to try and keep the blood sugars within a normal – or at least acceptable – range. Aiming for between 4 and 10mmol/l should be your goal and you will be able to keep a check on your child's blood sugars at any given moment by finger prick testing. This is fully explained in Chapter Four.

Types of Insulin

There are many different types of insulin which work in a variety of ways. However, they do fall into straight categories:

CLEAR INSULIN. As the name suggests, it is completely transparent. It is also called soluble, regular, short or quick acting. It begins to work shortly after it has been injected and continues working for up to eight to ten hours. It peaks, which means it is at its most effective, between two to four hours. As blood sugar levels are highest after food this clear insulin is the type that works, soon after it has been injected, on a main meal such as dinner. However, to prevent having to inject before every meal throughout the day there is:

CLOUDY INSULIN. This is opaque, looks thick and is sometimes called intermediate or slow acting. Once it has been injected it starts to work after about one to two hours. This type of insulin can work for as long as twenty-four hours but *usually* lasts for twelve to fourteen hours. Its peak is at six to eight hours. Therefore, when injected before breakfast it starts to work before lunch and peaks at the same time as the rise in blood sugar after lunch. It then continues to work as a background insulin and covers the afternoon snack and goes on working until the evening meal, before which another injection may be given. There are also cloudy insulins which are long-acting and can last up to thirty-six hours.

BI-PHASIC INSULIN. This is also cloudy in appearance and is a *fixed* mixture, whereas clear and cloudy come in separate bottles to be mixed if required. Bi-phasic insulin is a ready-mixed combination of the previous two, and comes in different ratios of clear to cloudy, such as 30/70 which is 30% clear and 70% cloudy. The amount of short-acting, clear insulin is always written first on the bottle.

A few years ago varying strengths of insulin were used in Britain and elsewhere, called U20, U40 and U80. This was a complicated system and has now been standardised in Britain and many other countries, to U100 strength only. However, some countries are not on this U100 system. Indeed many European countries only stock U40 insulin, which must be used *only* with U40 syringes. Before you go abroad, always check what strength insulin is used in the country you are going to, just in case you have an emergency while you are there, and need to use that country's insulin and syringes.

The insulin prescribed for your child will be designed specifically for her; the permutations are extremely flexible and can be changed if necessary to suit her needs. Some children use fixed mixtures. Some 'free-mix' their insulin (draw up clear and cloudy from different bottles). Some just use cloudy insulin, some clear. There are *no* hard and fast rules. Your doctor will advise you what to use.

Insulin is measured in units, so your child will inject however many units the doctor prescribes. It is important that your child has the correct amount of insulin to control her diabetes. This also applies to the number of injections your child may have; this could be just one or as many as four. However, although young children often start on just one injection before breakfast, the vast majority of children have two a day; one before breakfast and one before the evening meal. It is a common fear among parents that a child's diabetes is becoming 'worse' when the doctor suggests an increase in the number of injections. But this is not the case. The doctor is simply trying to control your child's diabetes in the best way possible and increasing her injections from, say, one to two, could actually make her lifestyle a lot more flexible.

Shortly after diagnosis you may find that your child's blood sugar levels are continually running low. She may be going through what is known as the 'Honeymoon Period'. For some unknown reason the beta cells seem to make one last effort to produce their own insulin. This can last for weeks or even months and your child will need very little insulin during this time. But this does not mean she is cured – once the Honeymoon Period is over her insulin requirements will increase and you will know this by her blood sugar results.

As your child's pancreas is no longer able to produce insulin, the idea of injecting it is to imitate the pancreas as far as possible. Because insulin is a hormone and not a manufactured drug no allergic reactions should occur (occasionally the preservative in a particular brand may cause a slight skin reaction, but should this happen a more suitable brand will be found). The one side effect from insulin replacement is *hypoglycaemia* – or low blood sugar – which is why the timing of food is so important in keeping blood sugar levels balanced.

Insulin should be injected twenty to thirty minutes before breakfast and also before the evening meal, if taken twice a day. If taken *more* than twenty to thirty minutes before the meal, the blood sugar will fall too low before the food has been absorbed and may even lead to a 'hypo' during or after the meal. If taken a short time before the meal the food may be absorbed and raise the blood sugar before the insulin has a chance to act. Sometimes, though, it is not always possible to inject twenty to thirty minutes before food. There is no definite way of knowing when the food will actually arrive on the table if you are not eating at home. In this case the injection should be taken when the food arrives. It is safer to inject immediately before the meal rather than too early, which might leave a large gap. It's not uncommon to *forget* the insulin until your child is half way through her meal or even when the meal is over! Don't panic – just take it the minute you remember.

Once injected the insulin will work the way it's designed to; peaking and falling during the day. But once injected it cannot be removed and that is why it is so important for your child to eat at regular intervals throughout the day.

Here's an example of how insulin is designed to balance with food. Suzy, aged seven, takes a mixture of clear and cloudy insulin before breakfast and before her evening meal. The clear insulin starts to work about the same time as breakfast is being absorbed into her bloodstream. It will peak to coincide with the rise in her blood sugar following breakfast and then continue to peak through the morning. At around this time, the cloudy insulin is beginning to work. If Suzy does not eat anything mid-morning, all that insulin in her bloodstream will cause her blood sugar level to fall too low for the body to cope with, so she should have a mid-morning snack.

At lunch time, the cloudy insulin is beginning to peak to coincide with the rise in blood sugar following lunch. This lasts through the afternoon so Suzy will again need a snack to stop her blood sugar level falling too low. Her next injection is taken twenty to thirty minutes before the evening meal. Once again, the clear insulin will begin to work at the same time as the evening meal is being absorbed into her bloodstream and peak to coincide with the rise in blood sugar after the meal. She will also need a snack at bedtime to prevent her blood sugar level falling too low during the night.

Syringes and Other Devices

All the basic items you need for the treatment of diabetes are available free on prescription. Nowadays, syringes are made from disposable plastic and the British Diabetic Association suggests the same one may be used up to five times before it becomes blunt. A blunt needle would be painful; in fact, you may find your child will not tolerate five injections with the same syringe. You do not need to clean the syringe; if you always replace the cap and keep it with your child's insulin, there will be no risk of infection. Syringes are available on prescription from your GP and come in sizes of one hundred units or fifty units. Make sure you check which syringe you have before you use it as the measurements are different. Each line on the hundred-unit syringe represents *two* units and each line on the fifty-unit syringe is *one* unit. There are also thirty-unit syringes available but you have to buy these from the chemist as they are not, at the time of writing, available on prescription. These are a particularly good size for little hands.

Syringes are used for either insulin that needs free-mixing or for pre-mixed insulin. The advantage of free-mixing is that the amount of clear or cloudy can be easily altered according to your child's blood sugar levels. It is also especially useful to free-mix if you want to give a bit extra clear, or short-acting, insulin to cover a party or big meal. However, some children find it fiddly to draw up and mix two insulins in one syringe and often find it far easier using a fixed mixture.

Pens

There are also pen injection devices. These are made of hardened plastic and look rather like cartridge pens (the nib is the needle and the ink is the insulin which comes in a cartridge). The cartridge lasts a few days, depending on your child's dose, and when the old one is empty you change it for a new one, just like an ordinary pen. You cannot free-mix using a pen, but there is a wide choice of ready-mixed insulins available. Some children prefer to use pens as they do not look anything like syringes and this can avoid embarrassment. Insulin pens are convenient to take when the child goes out. Unfortunately, pens are quite difficult for small children to manipulate, which may provide an excuse for a fuss when it comes to injection time. Incidentally, the needles are not available on prescription so you would have to pay for them.

Pumps

Another device for giving insulin is called an insulin infusion pump. This is a small device worn outside the body, either on a belt or shoulder holster. Inside the pump is the insulin which is expelled through a fine plastic tube. The tube is attached to the body (usually the stomach) by a small needle through which the insulin passes. The pump provides a continuous flow of insulin which the wearer can control and this is particularly useful at mealtimes. For some people with diabetes they are an advantage, but they are generally not considered suitable for children as the pump may become dislodged during the rough and tumble of everyday activities. However, pumps are not manufactured in Britain at present, but existing ones can be repaired, if necessary.

Whichever method you use to inject insulin it is a good idea to learn how to draw up insulin using a syringe, simply because you would be really stuck if your child lost or broke her pen device and you did not know how to give her insulin any other way.

First, let's look at drawing up one type of insulin only and then at mixing clear and cloudy insulins in the same syringe.

How to draw up insulin from one bottle only (see page 38)

a　　Check the expiry date on the bottle.

b　　Mix the insulin by rocking the bottle in your hands or tilting up and down. Do this *gently* to prevent air bubbles forming which could be difficult to get rid of.

c　　Take the syringe and pull back the plunger to draw air into it. Draw up the same amount of air as the dose of insulin your child is to have.

d　　With the bottle upright (so the needle does *not* touch the insulin which would create more bubbles) insert the needle through the rubber cap of the bottle and push the air in.

e　　Do not remove the needle but turn the bottle upside down and make sure the tip of the needle is covered by the insulin.

f　　Hold onto the bottle and the syringe. Try and hold the bottle steady, if it moves around too much this may bend the needle. Pull out the plunger, the insulin will be drawn into the syringe. Draw up a little more insulin than you need.

g　　Remove the syringe from the bottle and with the needle pointing upwards, gently tap the syringe and allow any air bubbles to rise to the top.

h　　Gently push the plunger to expel any air bubbles or any extra insulin. Make sure the top of the plunger in the syringe is in line with the amount of insulin your child is to have.

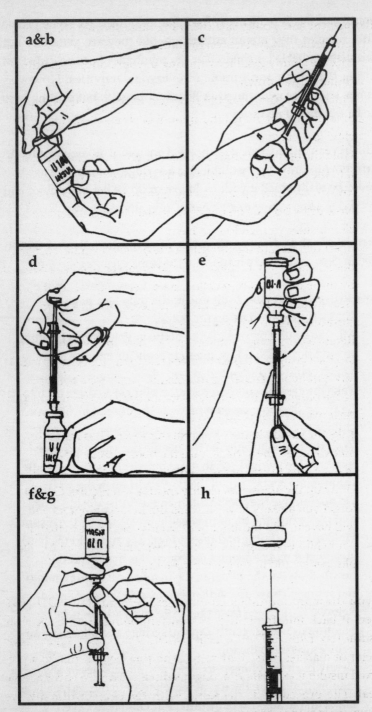

DRAWING UP INSULIN FROM ONE BOTTLE ONLY

Mixing clear and cloudy insulin in the same syringe

a   Check the expiry dates on the bottles.

b   Mix the cloudy insulin by rocking in your hands or gently tilting up and down.

c   Pull out the plunger of the syringe and draw up the same amount of air to match the amount of *cloudy* insulin your child is to have.

d   Hold the bottle of cloudy insulin upright. Push the syringe into the bottle and inject the air in. Remove the syringe. You do *not* draw up any cloudy insulin at this stage.

e   Now draw up the amount of air to match the amount of *clear* insulin your child is to have.

f   Inject this air into the upright bottle of clear insulin. Turn the bottle upside down, make sure the tip of the needle is covered by the insulin, and the bottle is held steady. Draw up the clear insulin, a little more than you need. You *always* draw clear insulin into the syringe first.

g   Remove the syringe from the bottle. With the needle upright tap the syringe so the air bubbles rise to the top. Gently expel any air bubbles and any extra insulin. Make sure the top of the plunger in the syringe is in line with the amount of clear insulin your child is to have.

h   Take the cloudy bottle of insulin (make sure it is properly mixed), insert the syringe, turn the bottle upside down, making sure the tip of the needle is covered by the insulin. Draw up the amount of cloudy insulin you require. Do not forget you already have clear insulin in the syringe so you will have to add the amount of cloudy insulin on to that; if your child is taking four units of clear and ten of cloudy, the plunger should be on the fourteen unit line.

If you draw up too much cloudy insulin by mistake, DO NOT inject it back into the bottle, as you will be injecting back clear insulin too. DISCARD ALL THE INSULIN and start again. Your doctor or diabetes nurse may suggest adding clear insulin to a pre-mixed insulin if extra short-acting insulin is needed to cover a large meal. The procedure is the same, with the *clear* insulin always drawn up into the syringe first.

The diagram opposite shows you the areas where insulin can be injected. It is very important not to use the same place every time. Repeated injections in the same spot will cause the skin to become hard until eventually the insulin will not be absorbed properly. This can lead to fluctuating blood sugars, making diabetes difficult to control. It is a good idea to get your child into a routine. For example, Monday morning could be the right arm, Monday evening the left arm. Tuesday morning the right abdomen, Tuesday evening the left and so on. Perhaps your child could draw an outline of her body, marking the areas chosen for each day and pin it on her bedroom wall.

Insulin is absorbed at different rates depending where it is injected. It is absorbed most quickly from the abdomen, then the arms, then the thighs and buttocks. Vigorous exercise also speeds up the rate of absorption, so does heat. It is not wise to inject before your child has a bath or shower as heat makes the blood vessels dilate and the insulin will be absorbed quicker, causing the blood sugar level to fall and this could lead to a hypo. Also, take care in hot weather as you might need to inject nearer the meal time (see Chapter Nine which covers holidays).

Injecting

This can be traumatic for parent and child alike. If you have a phobia about needles and show your fear, your child will immediately sense this. You have to approach injections in a calm, rational manner. Remember that your child will have to inject for the rest of her life, so it is vital not to create anxiety which could remain with her for years to come. On the other hand, no one would suggest that you behave in a completely detached way; your child needs to feel you understand her emotions. 'I had always hated having injections myself,' one mother recalled, 'and the very thought of giving Jenny that first injection made me feel quite ill. It took all my strength, in fact! But the relief when we had achieved it was enormous. I carried on for about three weeks and then Jenny took over quite happily herself.'

You are not injecting into a vein, just into the fatty tissue under the skin, so the procedure is quite simple.

INJECTION SITES

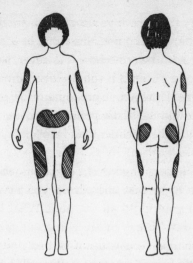

It really is amazing how some children take to giving their own injections. There is no right or wrong age for this; the average age seems to be around seven, yet some children as young as four or five will happily inject themselves (with their parents checking the dose of insulin before they inject). Please do not feel you have failed if you have an older child who will not inject; continue to encourage them. They are often motivated when they realise they could miss out on trips organised by school or clubs. The BDA organise children's holiday camps, and these are an excellent way of encouraging children to inject themselves. There is nothing like peer pressure to motivate a child! There will be other children at the camp doing their own injections and often being rewarded by a star system. A gold star can be won if all the injection sites have been used. You may be able to try this at home with younger children. Buy some paper stars from a stationery shop and award a different colour for each site used. Award a gold star when she has tried all the sites.

Any interest that your child shows in any part of the injection procedure should be encouraged. Some children are happy to push the plunger so long as you put in the needle. Egg them on with warm praise for any part they play and this will gradually encourage them to take responsibility and eventually take over. Don't worry – they will get there in the end! There can't be many older teenagers around who want mum or dad accompanying them on a date to give them an injection!

In the beginning try to take things slowly. You are both learning so you need to make time. Of course, this won't be easy, especially in the early morning rush before school. However, the injections do not only have to be a parent's responsibility. Any sensible family member can do this. How about grandma or an older brother or sister? One mother told us, 'Katie prefers her older sister to do the injections, apparently she's gentler than I am!'

Beware – if only one person gives the injections, that can be a real tie. If you happen to be that one person you may find yourself having to be with your child all the time. What happens if you want a couple of days' break or are going out early and leaving someone else in charge? You will not be tied down if your child allows other people to inject her, or better still will do her own. She, too, will be free to enjoy the normal events of a child's life like going to stay the night with a friend, going on all-day outings or even having holidays away from you.

It is possible to suffer from 'needle-phobia' (a fear of needles) and if the person expected to give the injections has this problem things are going to be difficult. If someone else in the household can manage the injections so much the better. But try to get help from a psychologist (see Chapter Ten) to get you over this phobia as quickly as possible. 'I certainly had a fear of needles,' says eight year old Vanessa's mother. 'But so did Vanessa and there was no time to get help. I just had to get on with handling the needles as if it did not bother me. For weeks I felt drained of energy just trying to cope with the situation.'

The Technique

Try to be firm but kind. Have the syringe ready, make sure you have the right amount of insulin drawn up. There is no need to clean the skin with any spirit or swabs as this will eventually toughen it and make injections painful. Hold the syringe between your thumb and forefinger, like a dart. (If the child is very thin you may have to inject sideways, at 45 degrees into the skin.) If there is plenty of skin at the injection site you have chosen, then stretch the skin between the thumb and forefinger. If not, gently pinch the skin between the thumb and forefinger of your other hand to form a mound.

Push the needle into the skin – all the way to the hilt if you are using a short needle like those usually found on a plastic syringe. If you do happen to use a longer needle then push it in half way. If you do not insert the needle deep enough then a lump may form. Press the plunger. Pull out the needle. The less hesitant you are, the less painful it will be. The nerve endings are at the surface of the skin so the only prick your child will feel is when the tip of the needle pierces the skin. When the skin is pierced quickly and confidently it feels rather like a gnat bite. (Try it on yourself – *without the insulin!* – and you will get the idea.) If you notice a little insulin has leaked out, don't worry, this sometimes happens. You can seal off the hole by quickly pulling the skin to one side, but do not inject any more insulin as only a tiny amount will have been lost. If you accidentally hit a small blood vessel you may notice a spot of bleeding. This may cause some bruising but is harmless.

Once the first injection is over, you and your child will feel very relieved and you will both continue to gain confidence. You can also inject through clothes which can be pretty useful, particularly if you are out and don't want to join the queue to the toilet. Do remember, though, that jeans will blunt the needle more quickly. Of course there are some children who become distressed when they have their injections. One mother told us, 'I tried every trick in the book, yet there was nothing I could do to stop Georgina screaming from beginning to end. Injection time affected the whole family for several months but gradually things started to improve – she's fine now.'

If your child finds injections particularly painful or will not change her injection site because she finds a small patch on her leg most comfortable, there are a couple of things you can do to help. Some children tend to favour certain sites because repeated injections in one area cause the skin to become hard and lumpy and eventually the area becomes numb. Try putting ice on the area you are about to inject as this will make the skin less sensitive. You can make this into a game by using a packet of frozen peas or a frozen pizza; she could guess which frozen food was used while the injection goes in!

ANGLE OF INJECTION

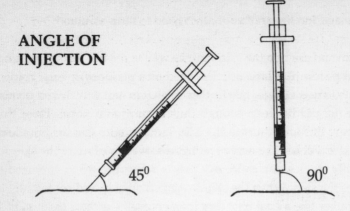

45^0

90^0

There are creams available on prescription which will temporarily numb the skin when applied to the area you are going to inject. But this is fairly impractical as the cream has to be applied at least half an hour before the injection. Also, your child may come to rely on it and you will run into problems if you forget to take it out with you and she needs her injection. This difficulty can also apply to the ice!

If your child really cannot bear seeing the needle being pushed into the skin, there are various other devices available. But once again, you would have to buy them. There is one gadget that looks like a tube or cylinder. You place the insulin-filled syringe into the 'tube' and hold it against the injection site. This device depresses the plunger without the syringe actually being seen – psychologically it might just help.

Practising injections on a soft toy such as a teddy and pointing out teddy's best injection sites may well help a young child find the whole situation more acceptable. Toy syringes can also be 'used' on dolls, teddies or friendly pets – but make sure the real syringe never finds its way into the toy medical set!

You may have heard about 'jet sprays'. These gadgets do not have a needle. But as the insulin enters the skin under a considerable amount of pressure they are not pain free, and they are extremely expensive to buy.

The British Diabetic Association advertises various injection devices in its magazine *Balance*, but that is not to say it always recommends their use. These devices may be appropriate for some people with diabetes and are certainly a godsend to some parents. But there is no escaping from the fact that insulin injections, for the time being anyway, are a normal part of having diabetes. It's not easy for anyone – child or adult – to accept that they have diabetes, but by accepting ordinary insulin injections and eventually seeing your child inject herself, you will be well on the way to adjusting to it.

Human Insulin

Human insulin, which is made from bacteria, is chemically identical to insulin found in the human pancreas. As it is a synthetic product manufactured under sterile conditions it is not possible for it to cause AIDS or any other infectious condition. Before Human insulin was derived, insulin was extracted from the pancreas of pigs or cattle. These insulins were chemically *not* the same as insulin from humans. As Human insulin is the same as the insulin humans normally produce, it would seem very reasonable that it is used. The BDA reports that approximately eight out of ten insulin-dependent diabetics now use Human insulin.

There have been reports that a small number of people with diabetes found their hypo symptoms altered since they changed from animal to Human insulin and there have been some problems. However, as your child will probably be started on Human insulin she will not experience a change-over. She will learn to recognise her hypo signs on Human insulin from the beginning, with no other experience to go by. If by any chance your child has been changed over from animal to Human insulin and you or she are not happy you should speak to your doctor. Animal insulin is still available and you may be able to change back. In reality, the number of people experiencing problems when changing from animal to Human insulin is tiny compared to the number of diabetics that there are.

What Hypos Are and How to Deal With Them

A 'hypo' is a short way of referring to a *hypoglycaemic attack*, or low blood sugar and hypos are the only real side effect of insulin. When the blood sugar drops below about 3mmol/l a hypo is likely to occur. In fact, many diabetics get early warning signs of an impending hypo before their sugars are very low.

Initially, the possibility of a hypo is the greatest fear of many parents. They may have heard of people with diabetes 'passing out' in the street or becoming unconscious. One mother told us that before her child experienced his first hypo her imagination ran riot. 'I had visions of Tom going hypo while crossing the road and getting run over.' She wasn't alone; so many parents expressed their fears. 'I imagined Emma lying on the floor, kind of paralysed and foaming at the mouth.' However, this is fear of the unknown which is only to be expected. Once a hypo has occurred and been successfully dealt with by you and your child, you are likely to feel less anxious and more confident that both of you will be able to recognise the symptoms next time. Sometimes hospital medical staff may deliberately induce a hypo by withholding food to show both you and the child what to expect and how to deal with it. Sometimes hypos happen for no apparent reason but they can usually be prevented.

There are three main reasons why your child could become hypo:
- a missed or delayed meal
- too much insulin
- extra exercise.

(Another reason is too much alcohol – be prepared for the future!)
So, to gain good control of the blood sugar level so that it is neither too low or too high there has to be a balance between food, insulin and exercise.

Children do not usually miss meals from choice but you should make sure that this *never* happens. Eating regularly with the right snacks between meals and before bed should prevent hypoglycaemia. There will be times when a meal is delayed and if possible this should be anticipated. An extra snack at the time that the meal should have been eaten will prevent the blood sugar going too low and keep it steady until the meal arrives.

If too much insulin is given by accident, this can usually be overcome by the child eating extra carbohydrate. For safety's sake you should contact your doctor or diabetes specialist nurse to let them know how much extra has been taken.

How Hypos Feel

The common symptoms of hypos are trembling, sweating and numbness or 'pins and needles' around the mouth. Your child might act as if drunk or confused, become weepy, or complain of blurred vision. Other symptoms are irritability, bad temper and irrationality. She might say she has a tummy ache or headache. She may also describe herself as feeling 'dizzy', 'funny' or 'wobbly'.

'My son goes as white as a sheet with big black rings under his eyes,' says one father. 'He says that he feels "wobbly" and wants to do a blood test. After a sweet fizzy drink and a couple of digestive biscuits he's dashing around in the normal way. We have encouraged him to speak up the minute he feels "wobbly" and we can sort him out before things go any further.'

Another mother described her daughter as 'very quiet and trance-like'. Other parents described symptoms of anger or clumsiness. All people with diabetes have their individual hypo symptoms which you will soon learn to recognise. If your child uses a word like 'funny' or 'wobbly' to describe her hypo at least she and your family will know what it means. One five year old even used the description 'magic'! Make sure her teachers, babysitters and anyone else she will be spending time with know her symptoms.

What to Do About Hypos

As soon as you or your child sense a hypo coming on you should act immediately. Give her something sugary to eat or drink such as:
- a couple of teaspoons of sugar in milk
- a glass of Lucozade or ordinary cola
- chocolate
- two teaspoons of honey.

If she carries glucose tablets, three should be enough. She will begin to feel better within a few minutes. If not, then give her some more. Once her symptoms have disappeared then she should have some starchy carbohydrate to prolong that raised sugar level as the effect of sugary carbohydrate does not last very long. If the sugar level falls again she will have another hypo and you will be back to square one. The majority of hypos can be caught in their very early stages and dealt with in a matter of moments. If your child is old enough to understand what to do by herself she should always carry glucose tablets and take them if the first signs of a hypo occur.

If your child's hypo becomes so advanced that she is confused or is too aggressive to take food or drink, don't use a glass to try and get fluid down her. Try rubbing sugary jam or honey inside her mouth with your finger. But beware – she may bite! The sugar will be absorbed through the lining of the cheek or swallowed with the saliva. A good idea is to use a glucose gel called *Hypostop* which comes in a plastic bottle with a spout. The gel can easily be squirted into the side of the mouth. Some parents find it very effective and they don't get their fingers bitten!

If your child does not have something sugary to raise her blood sugar level then the hypo will become advanced and she may become unconscious. Some children may even 'fit'. This can be frightening for you as a parent but if you know what to do you can manage the situation:

1   Make sure she is lying down (but not on her back).
2   Do not try to give her anything by mouth as she will not be capable of swallowing and could choke.
3   Make sure she does not hurt herself. Move any hard objects out of the way, i.e. chairs or tables.
4   Make sure she is warm and put a cover over her if she is not already in bed.
5   Try rubbing glucose gel onto the gums. If this does not work, give an injection of *Glucagon*. If you are unable to bring her round in 20 minutes (which is pretty unlikely), call an

ambulance. The ambulance staff will give glucose intravenously.

Glucagon

This is a hormone which works in the opposite way to insulin. When active it causes the liver to release its own supply of sugar into the body. Quick-acting glucagon for injecting is a solution which comes in a kit. The kit contains two small glass bottles, one with powder, the other with sterile water. It also comes with a plastic syringe. Draw up the water using the syringe, then inject the water into the bottle containing the powder. Shake the bottle to allow the powder to dissolve, then draw half the mixture back into the syringe (this is usually enough for a child). Glucagon is best injected under the skin. You can inject into the thigh, the upper arm, or the top outer quarter of the thigh. Pinch the skin and inject at a straight ninety-degree angle. Your child will start to come round in ten to twenty minutes. Once she is awake you can give a sweet drink followed by some starchy food, which should be given little and often. Don't be alarmed if she is sick as this often happens after glucagon is given. If your child does not come round in ten to twenty minutes, call your doctor as she may need glucose injected directly into a vein. Glucagon is available on prescription from your GP or hospital. It is a good idea to get hold of an out-of-date glucagon kit from your chemist or hospital pharmacy to practise with so if your child does experience a severe hypo you won't be all fingers and thumbs when you come to use it. Parents worry that frequent hypos – particularly like those we have just described – will impair a child's intelligence. Although hypos are better avoided, there is no need to become unduly concerned as there is no evidence of any brain damage arising from hypos. As far as physical damage is concerned, it is more dangerous to run high blood sugars (in an attempt to prevent hypos) as your child will be more at risk from complications of diabetes which can arise in later life (see Chapter Four).

Many parents have told us that they fear night-time hypos as they may be unaware of what is happening. Some children do cry out, often loudly and in a terrified manner and in this case a parent can respond. But what happens if you don't know your child is hypo? One mother said, 'I am worried sick that John will have a hypo during the night and I won't hear him. I am so afraid that he will become brain damaged or die.'

The majority of children wake up or cry in their sleep; some come to their parents complaining of their usual hypo symptoms. But even if they don't, they will *not* die or become brain damaged. This is because, once the body senses a low blood sugar, two things happen. Firstly, the body converts its stored starch into sugar. Secondly, the body's own supply of the hormone glucagon will rise and this in turn causes a release of sugar which is stored in the liver. The result of this is a rise in your child's blood sugar level and she will eventually come out of her hypo. If you find your child has high blood sugars in the morning which have nothing to do with what she has eaten the night before, this could be the result of a night-time hypo as all the sugar released by the body has not yet gone back to normal. Do *not* give extra insulin to bring the blood sugar level down, just give your child her normal dose. Extra insulin would probably cause another hypo. Ask yourself why it could have happened. Did she do a lot of strenuous exercise during the day and not have enough carbohydrate? (See Chapter Seven.) Did she miss her bedtime snack? Did she accidentally have too much insulin? If you cannot come up with an answer then your doctor or diabetes nurse may advise you to blood test your child during the night (around 2 am) to determine whether she is going hypo at night. If you do find her blood sugars are low and she has had a substantial bedtime snack, the evening insulin probably needs reducing.

As we explained before, it is quite possible to prevent hypos happening or at least, spot the early warnings. Many children never experience the kind of severe hypos that you may dread happening. It is up to you to train your child from the beginning of her diabetes to understand her body and respond quickly to familiar signs.

Incidentally, crafty children who enjoy the sweet tastes of their hypo-stoppers may feign their symptoms, but you have the technology to catch them out – the blood test . . .

Chapter 4

The Importance of Testing

'My confidence disappeared whenever Jenny had a high blood sugar – I've trained myself to ignore the odd "spikes" and deal calmly with changes that are needed . . .'

'I never let a day go by without at least one test. Whatever the results, they give me a feeling of security. I feel I'm in the driving seat . . .'

'I've noticed a definite growth pattern with Adam's blood sugar levels. They will be fine for weeks then suddenly go sky high and he seems to have become taller . . .'

Why Good Control Matters

Over the years doctors have realised that it's not enough to simply give insulin to people with diabetes and hope for the best. They now know it is also important to monitor the level of sugar in the blood and actually control it. This is, of course, mainly helped by insulin, but also by diet and exercise. Maintaining a normal blood sugar level is extremely important: if sugar levels remain high over many years, this may lead to damage of the nerve tissues and blood vessels around the body. This damage is usually referred to as 'diabetic complications'. You may hear of people whose eyesight has been affected, or of food and kidney problems. There will always be a jolly soul with some horror story to tell which will make you fret.

Please do not let yourself become anxious and depressed. It is important to remember that complications develop because of years of long-term poor control. Your child will *not* go blind because she has had a short period of high blood sugars. It's a fact that even ten years ago there was simply not the technology we have today to enable people with diabetes to monitor their blood sugars at home. These people would have had to wait months between visits to the clinic and even then the tests done there told them very little. The big breakthrough in diabetes management – indeed, the key to the future – has been day-to-day home monitoring.

It has been said that twenty-five per cent of people with insulin-dependent diabetes seem to be immune to any complications for some reason nobody quite understands. Researchers feel this is probably due to their genetic make-up. It is not conclusively proven yet but it does appear that avoiding wide swings in blood sugars and keeping them as near normal as possible will make someone with diabetes less likely to develop complications. However, something that may or may not happen in the future should *never* be used as a threat to your child. There is simply no point in worrying or dwelling on it.

Also remember that the regular screenings your child should have will pick up any problems if they do arise and then treatment can be carried out. Sensible home care like teaching your child that smoking is bad (as this also damages the blood vessels), taking a low fat diet and plenty of exercise will also go a long way towards minimising the risks. Do speak to your doctor or diabetes specialist nurse if you are worried, they will be able to give you the facts and reassure you.

How You Know What's Happening

Controlling diabetes not only helps to prevent complications but also enables your child to grow as he should: high blood sugars can stunt growth. Monitoring the sugar levels either by blood or urine testing will tell you how well controlled your child's diabetes is, on a daily basis. But beware! If your child feels well this is *not* an indication that the diabetes is under control and the blood sugar levels are below 10mmol/l. People with diabetes can feel perfectly well with raised blood sugar levels. Even if they do not have any symptoms, poor control can lead to complications. Monitoring sugar levels will also give you peace of mind and reassurance that all is well. If tests show sugar levels are too high you are in a position to act and get things right. Your child's test results will let you know if he is having the right amount of insulin. For instance, if he regularly has high blood sugar levels throughout the day, then he may require more insulin before breakfast. You would never have known about that unless you had been testing.

Testing also tells you what causes sugar levels to become too high or too low. For example a walk in the park is hardly likely to lower your child's blood sugar level, whereas riding a bike around the park may lower it considerably. You will then be able to anticipate events; the next time you are off for a bike ride, give your child a snack first (see Chapter Seven on Exercise).

Anticipating high or low blood sugars is an important part of diabetes care and you will soon learn to predict what will happen in certain situations so you will be able to keep things normal by altering insulin or diet. Sometimes, however, you may find high results for no apparent reason. These can be due to hormonal changes in the body. Discuss these phases – if and when they arise – with your doctor or diabetes nurse.

Urine or Blood – Which Test is Best?

The method of testing for sugar you are taught will depend on your clinic.

If there is too much sugar in the blood, i.e. more than 10mmol/l, sugar spills into the urine. Testing urine for sugar involves dipping a special paper strip into the urine. The pad on the end of the strip will change colour if there is sugar in the urine. You match the strip against a colour chart to determine how much sugar is present. The sugar in a urine test is measured in percentages (milligrams of sugar in 100 millilitres of urine). Any measure above 0% means that sugar has spilled over into the urine. If the strip does not change colour the result is 0%, or negative, which means that the blood sugar level is probably below 10mmol/l. The problem is that the test does not pinpoint the blood sugar level exactly – it could be 4mmol/l or 9mmol/l.

Urine testing is easier than blood testing, but not so efficient. Some children dislike the idea of testing something which is usually flushed down the toilet. They may actually prefer to prick their finger rather than do urine tests.

The point at which sugar crosses the 'threshold' from the blood to the kidneys and is then passed out in the urine is called the 'renal threshold'. Although the 'renal threshold' is generally around 10mmol/l, this can sometimes vary. Some diabetics can even show sugar in their urine when their blood sugar level is as low as 4mmol/l and this can make urine testing very misleading. The hospital or clinic may be able to tell you your child's 'renal threshold'.

Also, the urine test will be 'old news'. Urine in the bladder has probably been there for a couple of hours, so if the blood sugar level was high at a particular time, sugar will have spilled into the urine. By the time you do a urine test, your strip will show a positive colour change. But during the hour or so the urine was in the bladder your child could have been running around and his blood sugar level could have dropped, even causing him to become hypo. So, you would find a high urine test but low blood sugar symptoms at the same time. The way round this is to teach your child to empty the bladder, wait about half an hour, empty the bladder again and then do the test on this fresh urine. The result of this test will more likely correspond with a blood test. Basically, the aim is for all urine tests to be negative. The best time to test is before a meal, for example, before breakfast and before the evening meal. However, you may be asked to test after all food, as well, as this often provides useful information. If you are testing before a main meal, test *before* the insulin injection. If your child is unwell then you must test more frequently, as illness can cause a rise in blood sugar levels (see Chapter Nine). Your diabetes nurse will give you a book to write the results in. These results will show you certain times when your child's sugar level is too high or too low – then you can take action.

Blood Testing

The main advantage of blood testing is that it shows precisely what the blood sugar level is at the exact time you test; it is up-to-the-minute information. Many people find this very reassuring. You will even be able to catch your child out if he tells you he is hypo and blood test results prove otherwise! Your diabetes nurse will show you how to perform a blood test which involves pricking the finger using a small needle or 'lancet' especially designed for this purpose. You can buy automatic devices which will prick the skin with speed and the minimum amount of discomfort. It is also possible to take a spot of blood from the ear-lobe for testing.

The idea is to obtain a large enough drop of blood to cover a test pad found on the blood testing strip. There are several brands of blood testing strip available. Follow the directions given for the brand of strip you use. You will get your result in a matter of 30 seconds to 2 minutes, either by matching the colour on the pad to a colour chart on the bottle of strips, or by a computerised reading on a meter. There are a number of small electronic meters available for measuring blood sugar if you don't want to have to worry about matching colours, but these have to be paid for as they are not available on prescription in the UK. Children inevitably love meters, counting-down numbers and guessing results. However, if they are not used correctly they will give a false reading and you would be better off checking a colour chart visually. Consult your diabetes specialist nurse before you buy one and ask her to show you how the machine you want to buy works. Don't think you must have a meter. They are a luxury, *not* a necessity.

At the beginning you will be asked to test your child's blood sugar frequently. The results will tell you and the diabetes team if the insulin dose is right. The results also give you a good idea of what makes your child's sugar levels go up or down. Once some control

BLOOD TESTING

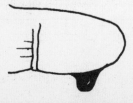 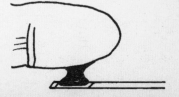

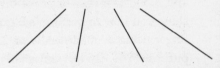

TESTED BLOOD GLUCOSE LEVELS
(in mmol/litre)

MONTH Feb		Before B/Fast	After B/Fast	Before Lunch	After Lunch	Before Dinner	Evening	Before Bed
Day	Date							
MON	1	3.9		15.0		12.5		9.0
	2	5.0						2.0
	3							8.5
	4	6.0				6.5		5.5
	5	5.2						17.0
SAT	6			15.0		12.5		
SUN	7			16.2		15.1		
	8	4.1				7.2		6.8
	9	2.0						4.1
	10	4.5				13.1		
	11					2.0		6.2
	12	6.1				7.0		8.2
SAT	13			5.2		6.8		
SUN	14							
	15	4.3				7.2		15.
	16							
	17	2.0						5.
	18	2.4				8.2		
	19	2.2						8.
SAT	20	5.6		6.1		4.5		
SUN	21							
	22	6.4						19.0
	23	5.0						6.0
	24							22.
	25	7.2				12.0		5.6
	26					2.0		8.2
	27			8.0		5.0		9.0
	28	6.0		4.0		15.6		6.5
	29							
	30							
	31							

INSULIN DOSE GIVEN

TYPE OF INSULIN USED

e.g. 30% solution insulin (fast acting),
70% Isophane (intermediate/slow acting)

INSULIN		Pre-mix 30/70 COMMENTS
AM	PM	REACTIONS, MEDICATION, ILLNESS, ETC.
14	10	Off school with cold.
		Played with friend late p.m.
		Ate large cake for afternoon tea
		Sugars high: watched TV +
		no activity all weekend.
		Felt hypo before breakfast.
		Ate chocolate on way home.
		Hypo after school.
16	10	Raised a.m. dose for inactive
		weekends — weather bad.
14	10	Too much afternoon tea?
		Low before breakfast.
		Low again before breakfast.
14	9	Decide to lower evening dose.
16	9	Bad weather again, watched TV.
		No idea why high!
		Birthday party — ate too much!
		Felt hypo after school — not much lunch
16	9	A good day!
		High pre-tea, had big lunch.

has been established, you can test less frequently; perhaps once a day at varying times, or three to four times a day twice a week. The aim is for the blood sugar levels to fall between 4 and 10mmol/l. Don't forget, testing should be increased if your child is unwell, or if he is doing something out of the ordinary, like extra exercise, or when you go away on holiday.

Try to make the testing your child's responsibility, show him where to write the numbers and encourage him to take an interest. There is usually a space for comments, so fill this in if anything strange happens or if something has gone particularly well. The results will soon give you a pattern of blood sugar levels over the days and weeks. Depending on the highs and lows, insulin or diet can be altered accordingly. You may find yourself elated at good blood sugar results and despairing at high ones – and sometimes they hit the roof – but try not to treat them as exam results. They are no reason for rebuke! Try not to over-test; just follow the clinic's advice, otherwise your child will get very fed up with pricking his finger!

Try and treat blood tests as casually as injections. Don't make a point of calling your child in to do a finger prick if he is in the middle of playing as this will simply annoy him. If the test is due before a meal ask him to do it between washing his hands and sitting down to eat.

Getting your child to perform his own blood tests can be hard work; they often cause more refusals than injections do! They seem to be a real chore for some children, so it helps to get into a routine. If you test daily, your child will get used to the times and they will become part of his life. If you test on certain days, try not to deviate. You can even make testing into a game; have a sportsman's bet on the result! It's worth encouraging your child to perform his own blood tests but make sure he carries them out correctly. If a younger child refuses to prick his own finger then just show him how to put the blood on the strip until he takes over; or take it in turns to prick the finger and to get him used to the idea. Older children should be able to do this test without supervision – but it's worth keeping an eye on them as it's not unknown for record books to be filled in without the tests actually being done! This applies to urine tests too.

It's easy to see why children (and adults) write in bogus blood sugar results; they either can't be bothered to test or they want a pat on the back from the diabetes team and from you. If you suspect results are being made up, investigate! If blood sugars are being wrongly recorded and are actually high, problems could build up for the future. If you find out your child is not testing, try not to get angry. Tell him you understand that testing can sometimes be a nuisance, but it's in his interests to stay as fit as possible. If tests are being done but the results are made to look better than they really are, explain to your child that he is only cheating himself and that insulin and diet can be altered to get *genuinely* good results.

What to Do with 'Highs' and 'Lows'

Do not alter the insulin dose on the basis of one odd result, if the rest of the tests are fine. First of all try and work out why it may have happened. If your child shows a high reading could it be something sweet he has eaten that you don't know about? Encourage him not to hide anything from you and explain that it's important to find the reason for a high test. Did he have his insulin? Has he had a hypo and eaten a lot of glucose to recover? He may also have a high blood sugar after a hypo (as we explained in Chapter Three) because the liver releases stored sugar when the blood sugar level becomes really low. If you do find he has a high blood sugar about the same time every day, not accounted for by any of the above reasons, the insulin will need increasing. (Remember, though, the test shows how the *previous* injection worked.) If tests are repeatedly low, with lots of hypos, then the insulin will need reducing; or perhaps an increase in food or snacks is needed.

For example, if your child is on a mixture of clear and cloudy insulin and his sugar levels are high before lunch and supper the *morning* dose needs increasing. If before bed and pre-breakfast tests are high then it's the *evening* dose of insulin that needs increasing. If your child is only on one injection per day, the doctor or diabetes nurse will probably suggest a second insulin injection in the evening. Don't let this upset you – things have not become worse – it is simply the best way of controlling your child's diabetes.

Several parents have voiced their irritation at people asking: 'How severely has your child got diabetes?' There's no such thing as mild or severe diabetes. You either have it or you don't. The question they should be asking is: 'How well controlled is it?'

Because there are so many permutations to insulin mixtures (free-mixes or fixed mixtures), it is too complicated to go into every aspect of adjusting them here. The best action you can take is to ask the medical experts for advice until you are completely confident about adjusting insulin on your own. Please believe it, you will get there!

If your child's blood sugars are high in the morning (but low or normal at bedtime) there is a chance his blood sugar level is dropping during the night and he may be having hypos, causing the liver to release its store of sugar. Instead of needing more insulin to counteract the morning 'high', he actually needs to be given *less* insulin in the evening. You can find out whether this is happening by doing a blood test at around two or three in the morning. Let him know what you will be doing so as not to give him a fright. If he does wake up he will almost certainly go straight back to sleep.

Inevitably, parents are often unsure how much to increase or decrease the insulin, and there is no easy answer. The amount will vary according to your child's age, size and how active he is. Discuss this with your doctor or diabetes nurse, but be assured that it should be quite safe to increase or decrease the insulin by one unit about every three days. Sometimes there are no apparent reasons for high sugar levels; growth spurts coupled with hormone changes may be the culprit. Once the right insulin dose has been found your child should thrive and grow, making up for lost time!

Long-Term Blood Tests

Every three to six months your hospital will perform either a *Glycosylated Haemoglobin* (HbA$_1$) or a *Fructosamine test*. These tests show your child's average blood sugar level over the past two to three months (HbA$_1$) or two to three weeks (Fructosamine). Blood tests which even out peaks and troughs to show an average blood glucose level over a period of time are extremely valuable because the day-to-day fluctuations cannot give a broad enough picture.

Whether your child is given an HbA_1 or Fructosamine depends entirely on the hospital he attends. Some hospitals use the Fructosamine as the test is less expensive to carry out. The HbA_1 is more widely used, and because the result is taken over months rather than two to three weeks, it gives a far broader picture.

The 'normal' range of results can vary from hospital to hospital. Do ask what the normal range is for your particular hospital and then you will understand these results. The medical team will recommend any necessary changes in treatment if they are outside the normal range. These tests show *average* results and *not* day-to-day variations which is why it is important to do home testing: after all, interpreting and acting on home results are the key to a good HbA_1 or Fructosamine, which in turn is the key to good health in the future.

Ketone Testing

When blood sugars are very high, ketones are often found in the urine. You test for ketones in the same way as you test for sugar in the urine. After wetting a ketone strip in urine you match the pad against the colour chart on the side of the bottle. At the beginning you will test for ketones frequently but once things settle down you only need to test if your child's blood sugar level is above 17mmol/l or urine tests are two per cent for two consecutive readings. It is also very important to test for ketones if your child is ill or vomiting (see Chapter Nine).

Whenever you are apprehensive about how you should react to high or low sugar levels, speak to your doctor or diabetes nurse. You may be reluctant to alter insulin or make decisions on your own at first but you will be surprised at how quickly you gain confidence. Every time you alter treatment, tell your child what is happening and why. Sooner or later he will be independent of you and take over the management of his diabetes. The more knowledge he has, the better the job he will make of it!

Chapter 5

The First Few Weeks

'It will be difficult not to sit around feeling sorry for your child – or yourself . . .'

'Get yourself organised: write lists, timetables . . . anything that will clear your muddled mind . . .'

Thinking Positive

Now you are recovering from the initial shock of learning that your child is diabetic you must try to get on with life as a normal family, hard as it may seem at first. Try not to think of this as a traumatic problem to be overcome – think of it more as a series of hurdles, each one to be crossed as smoothly as possible.

Remember when your first baby was born? Remember how you felt when you brought it home from hospital? Did it feel strange; a long, dark tunnel perhaps, with no light at the end? Yet suddenly something clicked: you understood exactly what you were meant to be doing and everything fell into place like a jigsaw.

It may seem an odd analogy but diabetes puts you into a similar situation: to reach your goals (balancing insulin, food and exercise to reach a near-normal blood sugar) without letting such a major event completely disrupt your life.

You may say, 'It's not the same at all . . .' but think about it. A major disruption – granted, not a joyous one – comes along and you feel disorientated and muddled. Yet your aim is to carry on in as normal and sociable a way as possible. You want your child to be strong, healthy and to do everything as well as or better than other kids can. This is definitely possible, but you must try to be positive right from the start. Think of this as a challenge – one you can win. You are going to help your child become a strong, independent individual *because* of her diabetes – not despite it.

The first thing you must realise is that fussing, treating your child like a semi-invalid and wrapping her in cotton wool is no good at all. A low-key approach is the best way to handle this child and you should strive for this from the beginning. Don't avoid telling her off for things you would have previously done or she will become thoroughly spoilt. Don't bribe her to do injections by offering prizes. You will soon run out of ideas – and money! She will also become the object of envy by brothers, sisters and friends . . . and singled out as 'different'.

However, it would be fair enough to treat hospital blood tests and long periods of waiting at the clinic with a special reward. One mother says: 'Julia was very good about doing her injections and I felt so overwhelmed with relief that my instinct was to constantly buy her anything she wanted out of sheer gratitude. Thankfully I stopped myself, limited presents to her stay in hospital. Once she was home I confined any treats to the occasional clinic visits . . . something like a new book to keep her occupied as we usually had to wait.'

Another tells us: 'Whenever we go for Harry's long-term blood test he asks if he can have his photo taken in a booth in the hospital foyer. I can't think there's anything wrong in that and to Harry it's a kind of symbol of his hospital visits. It's hardly what I'd describe as blackmail!'

Some hospitals reward children with stickers, badges or special plasters after HbA_1 or Fructosamine blood tests which usually, being intravenous, tend to cause more discomfort than finger pricks. Some clinics give children questionnaires (usually provided by an insulin manufacturing company) to test their knowledge on diabetes. Certificates and prizes may be awarded as an incentive for children to learn as much as possible about the condition.

Getting Organised

Once you have been given all your supplies for treating diabetes you must begin a system of storage that will enable you to find anything you need at any given moment. It's no use running out of blood testing strips and not being able to find the new ones. A plastic container (the size of a large ice-cream box) is ideal. Syringes, testing strips, lancets etc. can all be kept together. Some children like to keep their supplies in a lunchbox with their favourite TV character on the front. One boy chose Count Duckula, a cartoon duck based on Dracula, 'because Dracula was always taking people's blood . . .'. You will also need a small carrying case (some children use a 'bumbag') for supplies when going out. There is a lot of equipment on sale from specialist manufacturers. Some carrying cases are thermally insulated and come with their own mini ice-pack. However, anything that is the right size for your child or your handbag or pocket will do. Blood testing meters come in their own smart carrying cases which are usually simulated or real leather and look like a diary or slimline purse. You can get meters, automatic finger-prickers and insulin injectors all disguised as smart pens, so older children can have a blazer-pocket full of them.

Keep your supplies away from young children who may decide to play hospitals with real needles! Do check every so often that 'use-by dates' are still valid and top up stocks if they seem to be going down. Insulin should be stored in the fridge – away from the freezer compartment. But there is no need to keep the bottle currently in use cold. Insulin injected cold is very painful and it will stay stable at room temperature for a month.

When you are discarding a syringe use a 'safe-clip' (available on prescription) which will safely store hundreds of needles. Dispose of the remainder (and used lancets) in a large tin. Many local authorities now provide 'sharps disposal' boxes which are small plastic bins which they will collect when full and replace. Ring

your local town hall to find out if they offer this service, or ask
your GP.

Where to Get Everything

All children under the age of sixteen are exempt from prescription
charges in the UK. But people with diabetes of any age, throughout
their life, do not have to pay for *anything* prescribed under the
Health Service – surely a rare perk?

The basic equipment needed for the control and treatment of diabetes
is available on prescription. This includes insulin, syringes, blood
testing strips, urine testing strips, ketone strips, lancets and safe-clips
for needles. Some doctors may also prescribe *Hypostop*, a glucose gel
(see Chapter Three). You will have to buy anything regarded as a
non-necessity such as glucose-testing meters and automatic finger-
prickers but these are widely available from chemists or direct from
manufacturers. Like all electronic equipment, the price of meters is
coming down all the time especially when newer models are
introduced and the BDA magazine *Balance* will keep you informed of
special offers and new technology.

You may have problems obtaining insulin pens from your GP as
they are, as yet, not available on the NHS. But you can get these
free of charge from your diabetes nurse. She will also be able to
recommend blood glucose meters, show you examples and
perhaps even loan you one to help you to decide whether or not to
buy. If you can afford to buy a meter you will find them fast and
accurate (providing you follow the instructions carefully). Children
love anything computerised with buttons to press.

Your diabetes nurse will also give you the book in which you
record blood or urine test results.

Identification

Your child should always carry a card showing that she is
diabetic. These are available from the BDA or your diabetes clinic

and it's worth getting a supply of them as they are bound to become lost or dirty.

Identification jewellery is a good idea although some children are not too keen on wearing necklaces or bracelets. You may be able to persuade a reluctant child to wear one of a range of medallions available depicting a favourite sport. These look attractive and unscrew to reveal identification and medical details. There are various choices of activities including riding, swimming, football and windsurfing in a variety of metals ranging from stainless steel to gold. Other types of ID jewellery include bracelets (some contain a central emergency number where medical details are stored on computer) and 'dog-tags' with a simple inscription such as 'diabetic on insulin' which are said to be the favourite choice among teenagers.

Most high street jewellers stock identification jewellery. Or you can contact the BDA for manufacturers. The most popular makes are *SOS Talisman* and *Medic-Alert* – their symbols are known worldwide.

What to Take Out with You

When going out with your child for the day you will need a small kit of equipment in your handbag or, if she prefers, in her pocket or 'bumbag'. Glucose tablets are a must (and you should make her responsible for carrying them) as is insulin and a syringe (or pen), even if you imagine that you will be home in time for supper and the evening injection. You never know whether you will end up staying out for a meal and taking insulin along 'just in case' gives you the freedom to be spontaneous.

Some parents we talked to bemoaned the fact that they did not feel free to suddenly change their plans and go out to eat, for example. But why ever not? The time that you and your family are likely to feel hungry is around the time your diabetic child would be eating anyway, so if you are carrying her insulin you can cover her for the meal and not be inconvenienced by having to go home for injection time. If you always carry a spare 'kit' around with you there is no need to feel tied to your home – but write the date you took the insulin out of the fridge on the bottle and replace it after a month.

Keep a small supply of mini-bars or biscuits in the glove compartment of your car, pocket or handbag and you will be fully prepared for the unexpected. If meals are delayed and you think your child might be heading for a hypo, give her a snack to bridge the gap. If you are thinking what a hassle all this sounds it's worth remembering the spare bottles, nappies, toys, comforters and timing of feeds that you had to think about with a baby. All that paraphernalia takes up *far* more space!

Get into a Routine

Once you've got to grips with the treatment that your child will need now that she is diabetic you will find it easier than you first imagined to find a basic timetable for insulin and food. Then, you can work around the guidelines and allow your routine some flexibility.

But first you need a basic routine to work from. Children like a certain amount of regime, so fit injections and blood tests into your already established day.

Let's presume it's a school day and take breakfast time as a starting point. Say your family usually eats at 8 am. Bearing in mind that your child will have to wait twenty to thirty minutes before eating (to give the insulin time to absorb into the bloodstream) she should have the injection at about 7.30 am. Many parents prefer to do morning injections in the bedroom or bathroom rather than the kitchen so that food in the immediate area will not be a temptation. If your child is old enough to tell the time make sure she has a clock or watch to hand and ask her to come to you at 7.30 am. Have your supply box ready. If your child does not yet tell the time or has to be woken up for school then you will have to go to her. If she is making a fuss about injections you may need to allow extra time in order to keep breakfast on schedule, so bear that in mind.

The majority of children settle down to injections (even though it might take weeks at first) and do them quite naturally along with their morning ablutions. By the time your child has washed (not bathed, as the heat will make the insulin absorb too quickly – save baths for the evening), dressed herself and messed around as most children do, it will be time for breakfast.

After school, injections will be before the main evening meal so perhaps some homework or TV could fill the twenty to thirty minute gap before eating. Between the times of these injections you will be able to work out times for lunch and snacks (see Chapter Six, page 83) and times for finger-prick blood tests (see Chapter Four, page 58).

There is no reason to feel tied down by these injection times and mealtimes especially on weekends or holidays: they are moveable by an hour or two so you can carry on having a lie-in.

Help and Support

One of the first things you should do now that you are becoming better organised is to join the British Diabetic Association (or BDA).

Founded in 1934 by two people with diabetes, the famous author H.G. Wells and R.D. Lawrence, a doctor working in the diabetic unit of King's College Hospital, London, the BDA is now a massive organisation with hundreds of thousands of members. It gives help and advice to diabetics and their families, provides large amounts of funds for research and has spawned dozens of self-help groups around the country. In many other countries there are separate organisations for patients and professionals (such as doctors and nurses) but the BDA is quite unique in that it incorporates both these groups and their varying interests.

You will pay an annual membership subscription although for children the first year's membership is free. Naturally, donations are welcome. When you first join the BDA you will receive a Youth Pack (and School Pack if you request it) plus the news magazine

Balance which is bi-monthly. They will also send you a catalogue of books, leaflets, videos and products associated with diabetes such as the carrying cases we mentioned earlier. The BDA also organises family weekends, conferences, youth schemes and residential holiday camps for children.

How parents feel about joining a local support group depends entirely on the individual.

'I joined our local branch within days,' reports one mother. 'I had no contact with any other people concerned with diabetes and found talking to parents in the same boat a tremendous relief.'

Some were not so sure. 'I went to one or two meetings but found that we went over and over the same subjects again. I suppose it can be regarded as a sort of group-therapy but I didn't feel I needed that.'

Another mother joined her local group several months after her daughter developed diabetes. 'I already knew two people with children with diabetes who helped me tremendously. I could ring them up at any time and talk for hours about blood sugars, the carbohydrate content of various biscuits and my worries and fears. They gave me all the support I needed. Once I felt confident I went along to our local branch to see what was going on. I enjoyed the discussions and felt that I now had some knowledge to contribute. I didn't need the 'therapy'; I simply enjoyed joining in, which I'm not sure I could have done at first.'

Some parents are wary of 'labelling' their children by putting them into a 'group'. 'We all went swimming and the children with diabetes were to told to wear armbands. For the life of me I couldn't think why! I've always been against singling Billy out as 'different' and this seemed ridiculous. We didn't bother to go again.'

You may share this mother's sentiments and thus dismiss the idea of sending your child to a specialist diabetes camp. After all, once she is *au fait* with her injection and blood test regime there is no good reason why she cannot go to 'ordinary' holiday camps, especially with the responsible kind of people who run Girl Guide or Boy Scout camps. However, the majority of children who go to these BDA camps (from age five upwards) have a fantastic time of non-stop activity (fuelled by many chocolate bars) and are oblivious to any worries of being 'lumped together' as a special group. The children also learn from each other. A real bonus of these holidays is that they are run by doctors and nurses who specialise in diabetes and any child who goes to camp unwilling to do her own injections nearly always comes out proficient in the art! And, last but not least, these holidays allow you, the parent, a welcome break from the normal routine.

Whether or not you decide to involve your child with others who have diabetes, you should certainly register her as a member of the BDA for this will be your biggest link with the many developments in this field that are going on around the world.

Disability Living Allowance

You are entitled to apply for disability living allowance (formerly attendance allowance) provided by the Government. This is paid in a weekly sum, the amount of which is decided after your situation has been assessed. Although some parents are turned down and told that the child is perfectly healthy and does not need constant attendance, the majority of cases are awarded the allowance on the grounds that looking after a child with diabetes is recognised as an extra responsibility; at least, until the child is able to take the responsibility over for herself (often after the age of twelve but definitely at sixteen).

A number of parents have said that they have not considered applying for this allowance as they do not wish to think of diabetes as a disability or that the child is an invalid. They also point out that there are far more deserving causes for the allowance than their children. This may well be true, yet many diabetes nurses encourage parents to apply because they feel that the money can be saved and could be a real benefit to the child in the future especially in a household where having 'luxury' items such as meters or special holidays would be out of the question.

Letting Life Go On . . .

The first time your child is invited out for the day without you will seem like a huge hurdle. Your first reaction may well be to decline the invitation adding 'She's not quite ready . . . But try not to do this – the sooner you let your child get on with life, the better. Unless it is a really disorganised scheme which involves long periods without any chance of food, there is no good reason to decline. Obviously if the outing involves injection time you will have to be sure that the parent in charge is willing (and responsible enough) to take over for you. If your child injects herself so much the better and the parent will simply have to oversee that the correct dose is measured and injected. However, unless your child is on more than two injections a day the morning injection can be given at home as usual and, if your doctor or diabetes nurse agrees, the evening insulin can wait until the child returns (see Chapter Nine on Special Situations).

Your child's friends will now know that she has diabetes and their parents will doubtless be most concerned that they do everything correctly. Ask them for their proposed plan of action and give the times of your child's snacks and meals. Explain the need for extra sugar before anything really energetic (especially if they are going swimming) and tell them what to do if she feels hypo. Provide your child or the parent with hypo-stoppers (glucose tablets are the easiest to carry) and any snacks that you feel are necessary. You will be surprised how many people have some knowledge of diabetes.

Do let your child carry on with her life however concerned you feel at this first hurdle in the process of 'letting go'. Trust other adults to carry out your instructions, give them a contact number and reassure yourself that you (or your partner) can be reached by phone if you are needed. It's highly unlikely that you will be.

Once your child has been away from the safe environments of home and school she will feel confident about facing the outside world, and so will you. One more hurdle has been crossed.

Chapter 6

Diet: To Eat, or What to Eat?

'We all eat far healthier foods now and have low-calorie drinks as a matter of course . . .'

'Our diet was pretty healthy before – the children never had sugar on cereal or ate many sweets. So not much has changed for Paul . . .'

'The diabetic diet is an almost perfect diet as far as our family is concerned . . .'

Changes in Thinking

The most misunderstood area of diabetes is often what can or cannot be eaten. Parents who have previously had no close contact with diabetes may have vague ideas taken from recollections of someone they have known with the condition in the past. These memories will not help in their initial understanding of what their child will be able to eat.

As one mother told us: 'I remember a girl at school who was allowed nothing but salad. As my daughter regards salad as something you feed to the rabbit I was concerned that she would eat nothing.'

Another said: 'A lady sitting next to me on a plane journey had booked a diabetes meal which turned out to be an unappetising plate of cold meats. About half an hour later, she fainted.'

One father, having diabetes himself, recalls his childhood as eating huge hunks of carbohydrate-free cheese to 'fill up with'. He says now: 'I haven't been able to look at a piece of cheese since the low-fat diet became fashionable.'

The fact is that over the last two decades the idea of what a person with diabetes should or should not eat has done a complete about-turn. As we mentioned earlier, before insulin replacement was invented the only diet that would help a diabetic stay alive for any length of time was virtual starvation.

The first approach to diet after insulin came into use was complicated, and, as has since been proven, extremely unhealthy. Starchy and sugary carbohydrates were virtually banned, leaving mainly foods containing plenty of fat and protein (hence the aforementioned cheese!). But the high incidences of heart and kidney problems prompted a re-assessment.

After exhaustive studies it became clear that a diet containing plenty of high starchy carbohydrates and fibre actually helped control blood sugars and reduced fat levels which are said to lead to an increased risk of heart disease. Once day-to-day blood glucose monitoring became available it was apparent that this new diet plan helped the diabetic's control considerably. The reason many parents are so concerned initially about their child's diet is that they imagine he will never be able to eat his favourite foods again. They do not know that modern ideas have completely revolutionised the diabetic diet. Pasta, potatoes, baked beans, bread and vegetables are definitely in! If you have not already seen a dietitian you will probably be pleasantly surprised when you discover that your child will be eating virtually normally. The diabetic diet – if it has to be called that – is high-fibre, low-fat, low-sugar with plenty of carbohydrate. This is a food plan that is recommended as healthy eating for the whole population. If your child previously ate a *lot* of sugary foods then these will certainly have to be cut right down and replaced on many occasions with low-sugar substitutes or products containing artificial sweeteners. But this is far better for children's teeth and general health.

Chocolate and sweet biscuits are *not banned*. As you will see later in this chapter they can still be given at certain times – after a high-fibre meal or before exercise they are perfectly acceptable.

If you have ever been on weight-reducing diets you will have noticed that low or sugar-free substitutes for almost every kind of sweet food or drink are now available and most manufacturers clearly detail the nutritional food values of their product on the packaging. Unless you have been specifically asked to weigh quantities of food you will be able to tell at a glance what the carbohydrate content of a single biscuit, yoghurt etc. is. The carbohydrate or starch value of food is the most important detail that the diabetic must take into account but fat and fibre values should also be noted.

To help you further, the British Diabetic Association publish a book called *Countdown* which lists the carbohydrate values of many branded goods and convenience foods.

How Foods are Broken Down

There are three main types or groups of food which, along with the vitamins and minerals they contain, are necessary to make the body work properly. These groups are *carbohydrates, protein* and *fat*: some foods contain just one of these groups but in many foods the groups overlap. For example, milk contains carbohydrate, protein and fat. A very important component also found in foods containing carbohydrate is dietary fibre and over the last few decades this dietary fibre has been proven to be essential for good digestion of food and may also play a large part in preventing bowel disease. Some carbohydrates contain a particularly high percentage of fibre and it is these high-fibre foods which slow down the absorption of sugar into the bloodstream, thus helping to keep sugar levels under control. In the old-fashioned diabetic diet (high fat and protein, very little carbohydrate) fibre would hardly have featured, being found only in foods containing carbohydrates. As research has shown, high-fat levels are damaging to the heart and the body's blood vessel supply. It now seems obvious that many diseases (often fatal) could possibly have been prevented by the diet now recommended to diabetics and, indeed, the general population.

It's interesting that as long ago as the Second World War fibre was thought to have beneficial qualities for everybody – diabetics included. Between 1941 and 1954 it was compulsory to use high-fibre National Flour which contained a lot more roughage than refined white flour. One eminent doctor, Hugh Trowell, pointed out that even though sugar consumption was higher during the early 1950s than before the war, the death rate from diabetes fell quite dramatically until 1954 – the year that National Flour was no longer compulsory. Dr Trowell suggested on the basis of this and certain other factors that had come to his attention, that it was the lack of fibre rather than the excess of sugar in the diabetic diet which could be important in controlling blood sugar levels.

Understanding Carbohydrates

You need to understand what part the carbohydrate plays in the diet, for this is the food group which directly affects the blood sugar and therefore the treatment and control of diabetes.

Carbohydrates (CHO) provide energy and so are very important for our health. In fact, there are two types of carbohydrate – sugary and starchy – and it is the starchy variety that should play the main part in your child's diet. Sugary carbohydrates cause sharp rises in blood sugars and even though they are not forbidden you should keep the consumption of these to a minimum – perhaps for treats. Sugary foods often have to be used to treat hypoglycaemia (very low blood sugar) and this has been fully explained in Chapter Three. But when you do want to treat your child to a favourite chocolate bar or cake, best to give it at the end of a high-fibre main meal when the sugar content will be absorbed slowly.

Starchy Carbohydrates

The main sources of starchy carbohydrates are: bread, breakfast cereals, pasta, rice, potato, pulses (beans and lentils) and other cereal products including biscuits. Fruit and vegetables also contain some starchy carbohydrates.

Sugary Carbohydrates

All the foods that rot your teeth and contain plenty of calories to make you fat are in this list! Sugar, jam, honey, chocolates, sweet biscuits, cakes, sugar-coated breakfast cereal, tinned fruit in syrup, sweetened drinks and condensed milk. Nobody actually *needs* these foods to keep them healthy although plenty of children (and adults!) seem to crave very sweet things. If you make a big deal out of banning everything sweet from your child except when he's hypo he will bitterly resent his diabetes. He may also feign hypos if that's the only way he can have something sweet. If he will always accept fruit (which is naturally sweet because it contains its own sugar, fructose) instead of chocolate, so much the better. But children are only human (well, sometimes!) and unless they have never been particularly keen on sweet things they may crave them even more and become devious in their means of getting the 'forbidden foods' – if that's what you make them.

It is certainly best to avoid sweetened squashes and fizzy drinks as these are absorbed very quickly into the bloodstream and will raise the blood sugar rapidly. However, they are useful in a hypo situation. Also, very sugary boiled sweets, bubble gum, jelly-tots and so on are virtually total sugar. But with so many sugar-free drinks, chewing gum and other alternatives on the market you can get round the problem fairly easily. It's chocolate which is, perhaps, the greatest temptation for which no substitute may be acceptable.

What About Diabetic Products?

You probably know that there are special diabetic foods, some of which children actually like and will accept instead of ordinary varieties. However, these often contain a sweetener called *sorbitol* or *Fructose* which can lead to diarrhoea if eaten in large quantities. The products are also very high in fat and calories like thier ordinary counterparts. They are also very expensive. The British Diabetic

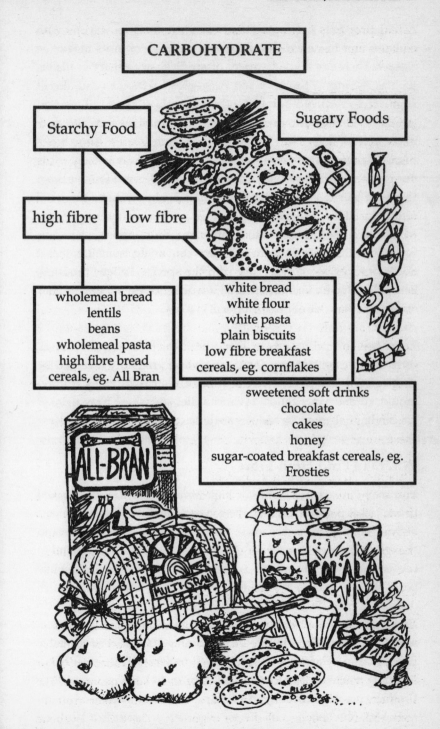

CARBOHYDRATE

Starchy Food

Sugary Foods

high fibre

low fibre

wholemeal bread
lentils
beans
wholemeal pasta
high fibre bread
cereals, eg. All Bran

white bread
white flour
white pasta
plain biscuits
low fibre breakfast
cereals, eg. cornflakes

sweetened soft drinks
chocolate
cakes
honey
sugar-coated breakfast cereals, eg.
Frosties

Association does not recommend these products for anyone with diabetes and has even stopped advertising them in its magazine *Balance*. There are a good variety of artificial sweeteners available, such as *Aspartame*, *Saccharin* and *Acesulphame potassium*; and also of sugar-free/reduced sugar products, such as jams, jellies and yoghurts. Low-calorie drinks are good alternatives too. You may have noticed sugar-free chocolate made from *Isomalt*. Isomalt is a sugar substitute which it may confuse you to learn is actually made from malt sugar but has only half the calories. Because Isomalt is not as sweet as sugar, foods containing it normally have artificial sweetener added. The rise in blood sugar from Isomalt is insignificant – but this is also the case with small amounts of ordinary chocolate. So the only real benefit from chocolate containing Isomalt is that it does not cause tooth decay. As with the special diabetic products, Isomalt can have a laxative effect so it would be best not to give your child more than one of these products in a day.

There are several brands of ice-lollies which have a very small carbohydrate content and these are always gratefully accepted by children. Alternatively, why not make your own using a lolly-mould kit and your child's favourite diet squash or fizzy drinks? He can have as many as he likes as these contain no carbohydrates.

Where to Find High-Fibre

You may already use plenty of high-fibre carbohydrates. If baked beans, jacket potatoes, corn-on-the-cob and wholemeal bread are part of your family's everyday menu then you are not going to have to change very much about your child's diet. If, however, you tend to use ordinary white bread, chips, cereals like Rice Crispies and white pasta, you can make a few changes without your child noticing much difference. If he dislikes brown wholemeal bread (some children do simply through the habit of always having white) there is a perfect alternative available: white bread containing 100 per cent vegetable fibre. It tastes delicious and he may well prefer it to the rather bland ordinary variety. Wholemeal pasta, bran flakes instead of Rice Crispies, potato skins instead of chips and wholegrain rice are all tasty high-fibre foods. Look out for *wholemeal* or *wholewheat* labels on biscuits and cereals – wheatmeal and wheatgerm are *not* high-fibre products. Wholemeal flour is a perfect replacement for white flour in cooking although disasters have been reported in the making of pancakes and Yorkshire pudding. This problem can be solved, however, by using half wholemeal and half white flour.

Most children like Weetabix and this should be encouraged. Puffed Wheat, Shredded Wheat and any cereal containing bran are good choices. If you child likes his cereal to taste sweet use one of the popular brands of artificial sweeteners such as 'Nutra-Sweet'. Raw or dried fruit such as raisins, sultanas and banana will also sweeten it. Cornflakes, Rice Crispies and other such unsweetened cereals can, of course, be used at times but sugared varieties like Frosties should be avoided. If he refuses to eat his breakfast without the Coco Pops he was used to, there is a compromise. Sprinkle a tablespoonful on top of a bowl of high-fibre cereal. The fibre will absorb the sugar when it is digested.

Many vegetables contain fibre but are so low in carbohydrate that they can be eaten freely.

Fruits vary in their carbohydrate content. Some fruits are very low in carbohydrate and can be eaten freely: strawberries, blackberries, raspberries and rhubarb are popular choices amongst children. Some are higher in fibre: bananas and apricots for example.

Pure fruit juices are fairly high in carbohydrates as their natural juice is concentrated. These do not contain fibre and are absorbed more quickly into the bloodstream. They are best used as a drink to accompany a meal rather than on their own – it is better to use diet squash. However, if you prefer to give your child natural fruit juice you could dilute a small amount with still or fizzy water for between-meal drinks.

Fat and Protein

Everyone needs fat in their daily diet to give energy and to store as energy reserves. It is also an important source of vitamins. But this is not to say we should eat an excessive amount of it. Fat has for some years been blamed as a major factor leading to heart disease in the Western world; a diet rich in dairy products and red meat was previously thought to be a symbol of wealth and good living. As modern research showed a high-fat diet led to premature death from cholesterol building up around the heart and clogging up arteries, in came the trend for low-fat diets and manufactured foods with a much reduced fat content. As people with diabetes seem to be at an increased risk of heart disease it makes good sense to keep to a low-fat diet to minimise this risk.

The exception to this rule, however, is in infancy. Babies and young children depend on a good fat supply for growing needs and energy. When they go on to cow's milk from breast or bottled baby milk (both contain fats) they should *not* be given skimmed or even semi-skimmed milk as neither would be adequate for their needs at that stage of their life. Semi-skimmed milk is not recommended for children under two years old and fully skimmed milk is not recommended until a child is over five. Children under five often find low-fat foods unpalatable and may refuse them altogether. At this young age, though, it's best not to worry about keeping a low-fat diet. By the time the child reaches primary school age his fat intake can be the same as an adult's. From five onwards you could use low-fat spreads, yoghurts, semi-skimmed milk, lean meat, reduced-fat cheeses and low-fat crisps. There are plenty of low-fat ice-creams on the market which taste just as pleasant as the 'rich-in-cream' varieties.

Please remember that this guide can only be very general and the dietitian who advises you at the hospital or clinic will tailor recommendations to the individual child. It is important that your child is seen regularly for monitoring. If the dietitian feels your under-five is overweight an early reduced-fat diet will probably be suggested.

Protein is found in meat, fish, eggs, dairy products, cereals, pulses, beans and peas. It provides growth and repair for cells and tissues in the body.

Many high-protein foods are also high in fat (red meat and cheese for example) and as there are low-fat varieties of these products it is fairly easy to keep to daily protein requirements on a low-fat diet. The amount of protein a diabetic child should have is no different from a non-diabetic. Incidentally, if your child is eating a well-balanced diet there is no need to give vitamin or mineral supplements.

Gaining too much weight is thought to worsen diabetic control so at each visit to the clinic your child will be weighed to make sure that he is within the normal limits for his age and height. Weight can be a problem in the child with diabetes simply because of the extra snacks he may have to eat to avoid hypos. This may be hindered by the fact that insulin helps store fat in the body. But please do not panic when your newly diagnosed child appears to suddenly fill out; he had probably lost some – if not a lot – of weight before he was found to have diabetes and is probably just going back to normal. The biggest mistake anxious parents make is giving unnecessary extra food to prevent hypos occurring, where they may not have done anyway. Your dietitian will recommend the amount of food your child is likely to need for each meal and snack. Try to keep to this. If hypos do occur you will be able to work out whether more carbohydrate was needed or whether the insulin dose should be reduced.

How the dietitian suggests you plan your child's eating pattern may vary from clinic to clinic. The two popular schools of thought are 'counting exchanges' and 'eating to appetite'.

Exchanges Explained

We use the term 'exchange' in the UK to describe *ten grams of carbohydrate*. They may sometimes be described as 'portions' or 'lines'. The idea of exchanges is not unlike that of a regular diet where items of similar values can be swapped around. For example, if your child's meal plan allows him four exchanges for breakfast he may want to have two slices of toast (one exchange each), a small bowl of cereal (one exchange) and a glass of fresh orange juice (one exchange). The next day he may prefer one slice of toast (one exchange), a larger bowl of cereal (two exchanges) with a small banana (one exchange). His drink could then be diet squash (no carbohydrate). The amount of exchanges the dietitian recommends for your child will be based on height, weight, age and lifestyle and should not be any more restricting than eating to appetite. However, the most common problem we found in our research was that as children's requirements changed they had often 'grown out' of their exchanges and were constantly hungry or hypo because allowances had not been made (often due to lack of attendance at the clinic) for their growing needs. All the more reason why the dietitian must be involved as part of the monitoring of your child's treatment.

If you are counting exchanges the task has been made simple by the labelling of carbohydrates on food packaging. Any food that is listed as containing nil or very few grams of carbohydrate can be eaten freely and not counted at all. Most parents report that they have become so familiar with carbohydrate value of foods that they are able to accurately guess the content of their child's meals.

The British Diabetic Association's guide *Countdown* is invaluable as it lists a wealth of shop-bought convenience products and everyday foods which are colour-coded according to their carbohydrate content. The BDA will also supply you with a foods values booklet to help you understand exchanges further. Incidentally, if a food is listed as having, say, thirteen grams of carbohydrate you count it as one exchange. This is safer than rounding it up to one and a half exchanges.

Eating to Appetite

Parents generally tend to be relieved when this system is suggested and it is the one being accepted more and more throughout the UK. The dietitian will want to know how much the child likes to eat at mealtimes and if she feels this is excessive then some changes may be suggested, such as substituting fruit for puddings which are significantly higher in carbohydrates. All children are different and the dietitian will assess their needs on an individual basis to maintain normal growth and weight.

Snacks tend to provide the biggest problem. A child who 'eats to appetite' may feel like two or three rather than just one biscuit. He may not need this amount of carbohydrate at that time; his blood sugars will go up and if three biscuits are eaten regularly he may gain too much weight. If you think your child is having too much in the way of snacks (or you are giving him too many, for fear of hypos) discuss this with your dietitian who will advise you. Some biscuits have a low carbohydrate content but are lacking in fibre, so only use these as treats after a high-fibre meal if your child has a special favourite.

The main difference between the two systems seems to be that once an exchange plan has been suggested, an insulin dose will be fixed to balance food requirements. With 'eating to appetite' the insulin may be gradually increased (almost by trial and error) to settle at the correct balance.

Snacks are of great importance because the diabetic on insulin needs to eat every 2–2½ hours to cope with peaks when the insulin is most active. Times will vary according to lifestyle and how many injections your child is having (see Chapter Three) but as a very general guide a regular meal pattern could go like this: breakfast – 8 am, morning snack – 10.30 am, lunch – 12.30 pm, afternoon snack – 3 pm, teatime – 5 pm, bedtime snack – 7 pm. This is not so different from the non-diabetic child except that the child with diabetes should *never* miss his snack.

Obviously this rough guide does not allow for your child's age or bedtime habits; if he is older he will have a later supper and bedtime, and so on. But as you can see, he will not be able to go for long periods of time without carbohydrate as the insulin will make his blood glucose drop and he will become hypo.

Hypo-Stoppers

However well your child's insulin and food intake is balanced there are times when he will become hypo – often for no good reason at all. If the child feels 'dizzy' or 'wobbly' you can usually bring forward a mealtime if you are nearing lunch, for instance. If not, you may be able to combat early warning signs with a sweet snack such as a chocolate biscuit. If this doesn't work and the hypo is progressing the main aim will now be to raise the blood sugar as quickly as possible. Sweet fizzy drinks such as non-diet cola or Lucozade will be rapidly absorbed into the bloodstream as will glucose tablets. Hypo-stoppers could be counted in carbohydrate grams because an unmeasured excess of sugar may send the blood glucose too high. It may then come crashing down again and possibly precipitate another hypo.

General recommendations for hypos are:
•10 grams of quick-acting carbohydrate, e.g. 50ml Lucozade; 100ml non-diet fizzy drink; 2 level teaspoons sugar; 2 level teaspoons honey, jam or syrup; 3 glucose tablets.

Follow this up with:
•10 grams of longer-acting starchy carbohydrate to stop sugar levels falling again, e.g. one slice of bread, a digestive biscuit or a small bowl of cereal.

If the child has become too drowsy or restless to accept food or drink you may have to resort to other methods (see Chapter Three which covers hypos in greater detail).

Sporting Snacks

As explained later, in Chapter Seven, covering extra exercise with carbohydrate is vital (it is possible to drop the insulin dose but most children would prefer something sweet and regard it as a treat). Your dietitian and diabetes nurse are the best people to advise you on how much and how often . . . again this all depends on the individual child, how strenuous the activity, how long she will be exercising and so on. Most parents like to give their children the treat of a small chocolate bar such as a mini Mars bar or Kit-Kat, whereas some prefer to give starchy fruit – bananas are ideal. A sweet drink alone should not be given unless the child actually becomes hypo during or after sport as the quick-acting sugar content of the drink cannot act for long enough to sustain the drop in blood sugar levels created by the exercise. Chocolate digestive biscuits, a piece of cake, a honey sandwich or a cereal bar are also good choices.

The Children's Choice

If your family diet has not previously borne any resemblance to the healthy eating plan we talked about earlier then now is the time to make changes. The changes need not be radical ones especially as the chances of your child suddenly accepting lentils or aduki beans are remote. It's more a matter of subtly introducing high-fibre, low-fat alternatives into your household.

Doctors are concerned that children with diabetes should live a normal life and not end up sneaking food they feel is 'forbidden'. Therefore it is not reasonable to stop all trips to McDonald's because you have decided to ban 'junk food'. You can still go out for treats to your child's favourite restaurants but it would be sensible to make these trips special occasions rather than the norm.

Try to change eating habits at home in an unobtrusive way. There are plenty of cookery books available that have good high-fibre, low-fat recipes. Some are specifically for diabetic children. But if you are not the kind of super-mum who can whip up a wholemeal pizza base and make it look and taste as delicious as the child's favourite supermarket variety (complete with white flour!) don't feel you have failed. Make compromises: try serving the pizza with a helping of baked beans or vegetables to provide fibre. Or try making a base with half wholemeal and half white flour. Wholemeal baps with grilled burgers, wholemeal breadcrumbs for 'Kentucky-style' chicken drumsticks and low-fat sausages are all good compromises you can try. Young children, especially, tend to stick rigidly to their favourite foods and often rebel against trying new tastes. They must eat, so the softly-softly approach is best. It is important, though, that your child is treated as other children and not singled out as 'different' by his eating habits.

We asked some diabetic children to tell us what they liked to eat and then invited a dietitian to comment on the suitability of their choice. We asked the children – who were all of normal height and weight for their ages – to describe meals on school days.

Harry, age nine years (packed lunch for school).
Breakfast: Apple juice, rice crispies or cornflakes, one bran muffin.
Mid-morning snack: Two plain biscuits.
Lunch: Raw carrot sticks, one small brown roll with corned beef.
Packet of cheese puffs. Small cereal bar, carton fresh juice.
Afternoon snack: Two biscuits, bag of crisps, slice soft-grain toast.
Supper: Two frankfurter sausages in bread rolls, baked potato,
peas or carrots, diet fromage frais.
Bedtime snack: One apple and one biscuit.

THE DIETITIAN SAYS:
'Generally, Harry's intake is very well balanced with regular meal
patterns. His carbohydrate intake is also fairly good but I would
like to see higher fibre choices: for example, at breakfast Branflakes
instead of Rice Crispies, wholemeal or wholewheat instead of
'brown' roll at lunch. Remember, brown or wheatgerm breads are
not wholewheat. Although cornflakes are not strictly high fibre
they do contain some fibre so are a better bet than Rice Crispies
which have virtually none. Harry's protein intake is fine; two good
portions of animal protein a day is sufficient for his needs. Nothing
is said about Harry's milk intake. Dairy foods are important for
calcium – essential for growing bones and teeth. Harry should be
having about one pint of milk a day (the semi-skimmed variety
would be best) or a little less milk but plenty of other dairy
products such as low-fat cheese and yoghurts.

'No need to worry about vitamin and minerals in Harry's diet. His
fruit and vegetable consumption is very good.'

Suzy, age seven years (eats school lunch provided).
Breakfast: Low-calorie squash, Weetabix and puffed wheat mix,
two slices of toasted high-fibre white bread with Marmite.
Mid-morning snack: One digestive biscuit.
Lunch: White bread roll, sausages and chips, apple.
Afternoon snack: Bag of crisps, low-calorie squash.
Supper: Jacket potato with grated cheese and baked beans, straw-

berries with ice-cream, two chocolate digestive biscuits, diet cola.
Bedtime snack: Reduced-sugar jam sandwich and fresh orange juice.

THE DIETITIAN SAYS:
'Once again, a good well-balanced meal pattern. Suzy starts well in the morning with a high-fibre breakfast – the high-fibre white bread is perfectly acceptable. Lunchtime is not so healthy as it is low in fibre and high in fat. It is difficult when only one day's intake is assessed as her general eating pattern needs to be taken into consideration. Perhaps substituting the white roll for wholemeal and a jacket potato for chips may be a suggestion although I realise this might be difficult at school. But for a one-off meal I would not be too anxious about this. Supper is well balanced. Having chocolate biscuits after a high-fibre meal is fine. Once again, I hope Suzy is having enough milk.'

Helen, age twelve years (eats school lunch provided).
Breakfast: Glass of milk, three slices of ordinary white bread with peanut butter, one banana.
Mid-morning snack: Bag of crisps and milk.
Lunch: Chicken salad, apple crumble.
Afternoon snack: Cheese sandwich, glass of milk, bag of crisps.
Supper: Fish fingers, peas and mashed potatoes, yoghurt, three rich tea biscuits, fruit salad in natural juice with single cream.
Bedtime snack: Bowl of shredded wheat and two digestive biscuits.

THE DIETITIAN SAYS:
'Again, Helen is having regular meals throughout the day to balance her insulin and that is very important. Her high-fibre carbohydrate is somewhat on the low side; having wholemeal bread and cereals, jacket potato with skins instead of mash and perhaps wholemeal biscuits at supper would increase her intake. She does have a good high fibre-rich bedtime snack, however.

'I would like her to have some high-fibre carbohydrate at lunchtime, perhaps a wholemeal roll or bread would suffice. It would slow down the absorption of the apple crumble which I assume is made with sugar. Her fat intake is a little on the high side – perhaps substituting the two packets of crisps a day for some fruit or a cereal bar and having low-fat yoghurt instead of ice-cream would be an idea. I would suggest Helen has a bit more fruit during the day. Although she has salad she needs more fruit and vegetables at lunch and supper to supply adequate vitamins and minerals.'

Eating Out

There are really no restrictions on what kind of restaurant you can take your child to, but it's worth knowing a little more about the kind of food you might be having. Before diabetes, you probably didn't pay that much attention to the carbohydrate values of Chinese or Indian foods for instance.

Here's a quick run-down on the different kinds of meal your child may like:

Indian: Usually particularly high-fibre as pulses (particularly lentils) may be used for making flour, and in vegetable dishes. Meat dishes such as tandoori chicken are carbohydrate-free but watch out for rich sauces which are often high in fat. Indian puddings are notoriously sweet but after a balanced high-fibre meal are acceptable.

Italian: A perfect choice . . . kids adore spaghetti bolognaise, ravioli and lasagna. If your child has chosen a dish with a very creamy sauce, discreetly ask the waiter not to pile it on! Watch the cream-laden puddings . . . don't deny his choice, try and compromise: one profiterole in a bowl of strawberries is a treat for anyone.

Chinese: There in not much carbohydrate in this kind of food apart from sweet sauces. But if you make sure he eats a good bowlful of rice (preferably the boiled variety) you shouldn't encounter hypos later. Try and share the portion of toffee bananas he may choose.

Greek: Pitta bread and rice must provide the carbohydrate as there isn't much else . . . dishes like moussaka are high in fat. Watch out for the tempting Turkish Delight with coffee . . . why not let him have one square and save the rest for hypos? If the pitta bread and rice is the wholemeal variety let him eat some more!

French: High in fat, rich puddings and not a favourite.

American: Up-market burger restaurants often provide jacket potatoes as an alternative to French fries. Massive syrup-laden ice-cream sundaes can be a problem. A dish of ice-cream without the sauce is a better bet unless you're going for a run in the park afterwards.

Fast Foods: Fine for treats and very convenient if you are out shopping and you need a quick blood-sugar boost at mealtimes. Bear in mind that pizzas, burgers, fries and milkshakes are pretty high in fat as well as carbohydrate. McDonald's provides a special leaflet: *For the customer with Diabetes*.

When eating out remember to order diet drinks and check with the waitress that the cola (or whatever) really *is* the diet variety. Many people can tell by one small sip, so you could check it yourself. You could even test it with a urine-testing strip, which will show if sugar is present in the liquid. The meal will be fine but your child can certainly do without the massive amount of sugar in ordinary sweetened drinks, unless he's feeling hypo when you arrive at the restaurant. If there are no actual diet drinks, go for pure orange juice which is usually available, or better still, mineral water.

If you are going out for a big meal it might be worth checking with your diabetes nurse whether you should increase your child's pre-meal insulin to compensate for the extra carbohydrates. Don't panic if you are on the exchange system and want to know how many grams are in the meal. With experience you will have a pretty good idea just by looking at it. Try not to become over-fussy and remove food from your child's plate because you think it's too much . . . it's his treat, remember!

While we're on the subject of treats, you will find that the majority of diabetes medical staff are most concerned that your child be brought up as normal and that means allowing him to 'let rip' at birthday parties, Christmas and other special occasions. If he is going to a party it might be worth asking the hostess (or rather the hostess's mother) if diet drinks will be provided. You will find that many families have diet drinks as a matter of course these days but if not, send a couple of cans of diet cola along with the child. He'll be too busy enjoying a free rein on the iced buns to mind about that small detail. Also remember that children's parties from toddler through to teenager inevitably involve lots of rushing around, musical bumps or disco-dancing so the iced buns and sweets will stop the drop in blood sugars as he uses up extra energy. Do make sure that the party mother knows she has a diabetic guest and explain that in the event of him feeling hypo he should be given something sweet immediately. The chances of this happening are, of course, pretty slim as your child will be making sure he hoovers up all the goodies he can lay his hands on!

Just to Prove How Much Things have Changed . . .

To end this chapter you may be interested to hear what this lady, now in her forties, has to say about her experience of growing up with diabetes:

'I developed diabetes in the 1950s at the age of nine and there was no way I could ever feel normal. This was not because of the injections – just the terribly restricted diet. Everything with starch had to be weighed and taken in tiny quantities. My Sunday roast consisted of a plateful of fatty red meat and cabbage with two very small potatoes. I could rarely have anything sweet unless I felt hypo and then it was always sugar lumps which I carried round with me. If I was bored at school I would transform my six sugar lumps into poker dice with a fountain pen so when I felt hypo and had to eat them, down went the ink as well! My blood sugars were often low from the restricted amount of carbohydrate and my weight soared because I ate so much fatty food . . . cheese was my staple dessert. I can't believe how much things have changed – I'm certainly making the most of the diet now. I'd never say it was lucky to be diabetic but it's certainly more fortunate to be a child with the condition now than it was when my generation was young. At least they can feel one of the crowd.'

Chapter 7

Exercise, Sport and Running Around

'Paul was never that interested in football before becoming diabetic. Now he's captain of the school team and hopes to play for the county . . .'

'I only find Suzy's blood sugars difficult to control when she's not running around . . .'

'Having a diabetic child has made the whole family get fit and become exercise-conscious. We've taken up sports we never knew existed . . .'

Exercise – the Big Balancing Act

Controlling blood sugar levels in diabetes is rather like juggling three balls: insulin, food and exercise. With experience you will find yourself able to juggle two balls relatively comfortably; insulin and food. The reason exercise, the third ball, often falls down is due to its variability.

Adults are usually settled in their day-to-day activities simply because their time is mostly taken up with work, study or domestic life. They usually know in advance when they are going to play tennis or have a swim. Adults rarely throw themselves into a spontaneous hundred-yard dash just for the hell of it or suddenly decide to play Indiana Jones and climb every tree in the park. Yet that's exactly what children do when you're least expecting it. Far from discouraging your diabetic child from joining in with the hectic games her friends are playing, you should give her every opportunity. Exercise is particularly beneficial for diabetics. It helps keep blood sugars and weight under control and is also good for the circulation. But you need to take precautions.

When we exercise, insulin in the body converts sugar, stored in the muscles, into energy. In diabetics, however, exercise causes the sugar stores to be burned up more quickly than they can be replaced by the liver: blood sugar levels will drop, resulting in a hypo.

There are two ways of dealing with this problem: eat more carbohydrate or take less insulin. If your child has a regular sport which is predictable in the amount of time taken and energy expended, then by trial and error (doing finger-prick tests before and after) you will be able to cut down her insulin beforehand and she will need less (or even no) extra carbohydrate.

However, most children prefer to eat the extra carbohydrate. It gives them the opportunity to eat their favourite sweets or chocolate. This type of carbohydrate is absorbed quickly and is suitable for short amounts of exercise, or exercise that has not been planned ahead. For example, your child could have a mini Mars bar before a scheduled games lesson. But if she is likely to be exercising for a long time, or the activity is particularly strenuous, she should have something longer lasting and starchy such as a cereal bar or small sandwich. This will not be absorbed as quickly and will keep her blood sugar stable for the duration. It is also a good idea to have some more starchy carbohydrate after strenuous exercise. Even then, you may find that she has a hypo sometime later, perhaps during the evening or night. A larger than normal bedtime snack can usually prevent this happening.

It is important to know that exercise can have this effect but don't be afraid to let your child tackle any sport or physical activity she enjoys. Exercise is good and it's fun! If you are concerned you can always do blood tests to give an instant picture of what effect it has had on your child and what adjustments you could make to food or insulin. It's always best to check with your doctor or diabetes nurse if you are not feeling confident about what to do, but it's usually preferable to let children work out on food.

Incidentally, while it's always beneficial to take exercise to help lower sugar levels, never think that it will work in the place of insulin and thus be tempted to miss out your child's injections. Unfortunately, diabetes does not work like that!

Highs and Lows of Exercise

It's pretty easy to get into a snack routine at school simply because PE sessions are set to a timetable and rarely last more than forty minutes. Most children find a mini Mars bar gets them through. Extended or indefinite periods of strenuous activity may need to be worked out, again by trial and error and – if possible – blood tests afterwards. Your child should always carry glucose tablets or have a bottle of sweet fizzy drink handy in case she feels hypo during the session. It may sound complicated, but you'll be surprised how quickly your child finds out what's right for her.

Younger children should always be supervised and the adult in charge ready with extra glucose should the need arise. Always err on the side of caution and have mini-bars handy for that walk in the park which somehow turns into a wild game of chase, but don't become so anxious that you must relentlessly feed your child 'just in case she hypos'. Give her some glucose at the start of her play session and rely on her or your own judgement to tell you when she's beginning to flag and needs the extra supply of energy.

Another thing that happens when we exercise is that the hormone *adrenaline* blocks the body's supply of insulin. If there is not enough insulin circulating in the body in the first place there will be nothing to work on the glucose. As we mentioned previously, in a diabetic the exercise itself is not enough to control the blood sugar. If you find your child's blood sugar levels *high* after exercise, this is a sign that she has not had enough insulin. 'Highs' may happen if you have cut down your child's insulin dose in anticipation of the exercise, or she is simply not having enough. If this happens, check with your doctor or diabetes nurse about the amount of insulin the child needs.

Sports and Other Energetic Pastimes

You may be worried that some particularly strenuous activities are unsuitable for your child. This is rarely the case as there are very few sports from which diabetics are discouraged. Scuba-diving, motor racing and parachuting are the only real no-go areas and even these should be judged individually.

Be assured that in other areas diabetes is no handicap: there are many sportsmen and women with diabetes who have reached the top in many sports. There are also many marathon runners with diabetes who start and finish their races *and* can manage their blood glucose levels!

Don't worry about any activity at school: your child will be able to carry on with everything as before. Obviously, some extra supervision will be required but (as you will see in Chapter Eight on School) this is not likely to be a problem. Obviously swimming can be potentially dangerous should a hypo occur, but as long as your child is never left unsupervised, and you impress on her the importance of getting out of the pool or sea if she feels a hypo coming on, there is no need to be anxious. Again, make sure the glucose supply is always handy and if she is invited to go swimming with friends make sure the adult in charge knows all the facts and understands that your child must not be left to swim alone.

Skiing, wind-surfing, horse-riding and bicycling are among a huge range of sports that your child can continue (or begin!) to enjoy. In fact, it would be a good idea to get her interested in something energetic (with a good social life as a sideline) that can be enjoyed into the teenage years. Many teenagers tend to give up exercise in favour of being a 'couch potato'. Lying in front of the television or in bed is *not* good for blood sugars and many parents find their child with diabetes has far higher blood sugar levels at weekends or in school holidays simply from lounging around the house with no energy being used. If you find this happens, ask your doctor or diabetes nurse for advice; you may need to increase the insulin dose for sedentary days especially if your child is 'allergic' to exercise.

Several mothers report quite a high increase of insulin is needed at weekends. One told us: 'Suzy's sugar levels are off the scale if she watches children's TV on a Saturday morning. We have to give her almost a quarter more of her pre-breakfast insulin to keep them normal.'

If you do increase insulin thinking that your child will be virtually immobile all day, only to find that her friends come round to play ballgames in the back garden, give everyone a bar of chocolate and let them get on with it!

Allowing for the Less Obvious . . .

If your child belongs to the Brownies, Beavers, Cubs or goes to any other kind of children's club, allow for the energetic games that will no doubt be going on. Many of these sessions start in the early evening, so if she has just finished tea she probably won't need extra glucose. However, follow the rule of supplying the adults in charge with glucose tablets and tell them the facts. If your child arrives home with a low blood sugar level, next time you send her, give her an extra snack to take. The same applies to any form of dance class, especially disco or country dancing when the pace is particularly frenetic. Bear this in mind at school, too, when discussing extra snacks with teachers. A Scottish reel can be far more strenuous than a game of cricket!

Chapter 8

Going Back to School

'I felt terrible when I left Adam on his first day back. I imagined I'd be seeing him that evening in hospital . . .'

'I sat at home waiting for the phone to ring to say that Gemma was having a hypo and could I rush over to help . . .'

'My husband and I crept round the back of the playground and looked through the fence at breaktime to see if Tommy had collapsed. But there he was, in the middle of a rugby scrum looking happier than he had done for months . . .'

Educating the Teachers

It will seem very strange when you first send your child back to school. It's only natural to feel anxious and protective while you worry about hypos, what he is or is not eating, and how he will feel amongst his non-diabetes friends. On top of that you will be apprehensive about how the school is going to cope with what they might view as a 'problem'. Your job is to make sure the school staff realise that having a child with diabetes is *not* a problem and will not be one as long as they understand what diabetes is and how to deal with situations should they arise.

If he has been in hospital and away from school for a period of time, returning to the classroom and the bustle of school life may be worrying for your child as well. If he has been treated as an out-patient then hardly any time may have been taken off and the routine barely interrupted. Either way, if you let him see how anxious you are feeling about letting him go it can have a detrimental effect. Do try to take things in your stride and allay any fears that *he* may have. If there are none, don't put yours in his head. The younger the child is, the less likely he will be to worry. If he has been unhappy at school previously this will simply be another good excuse for a fuss. An older child – especially one at secondary school who is expected to be in charge of his routine – may be more disorientated and bothered. Try to be reassuring.

Before your child returns to school you need to speak to the headteacher, his class teacher and the games staff. Find out if there are any other diabetic children in the school, because if there are, the task will be easier as, hopefully, the staff will know all about it. It's likely, however, that your child will be the only pupil with diabetes the staff have encountered so it's extremely important for you to give them full information about what diabetes is and how the routine works.

You may find that your diabetes nurse is willing to go along to the school and explain everything to the teachers (and the pupils if that's how you want to tackle it). If she cannot do this or is unwilling, contact the British Diabetic Association who will help. The BDA also provide a *School Pack* which includes information on everything including personalised 'hypo charts' that can be pinned up on staff room notice boards. Once the teachers know what is required they will be able to look after your child in a responsible way. If any member of staff is unhelpful or acts irresponsibly, you should take the matter up with the Head or perhaps review your choice of school.

Basically, the staff need to be assured that it is not dangerous having a child with diabetes in the class, that he will not come to any harm and will be able to join in totally with the other pupils as long as basic guidelines are followed. Some parents we talked to had come across problems, mainly concerned with meals, snacks and hypos which we will cover in more detail later in this chapter. However, the majority of parents have found staff to be helpful and kind. School life has carried on in much the same way as before.

Once your child's teacher understands the situation it would be a good idea for the teacher to explain it to the class providing your child is happy about this. To smooth over any resentment that may occur over extra snacks being eaten – chocolate before sport and so on – a full explanation should be given to the other children, with a reminder that the child with diabetes cannot eat sweets in the quantities and at all the times that his class-mates may. Injections and blood tests should also be explained thus making others aware of what's going on in case these have to be done at school. The thought of their class-mate having injections may well make some pupils feel less resentful about those snacks, too.

Encourage your child to talk openly about his diabetes and not to feel it is something to hide. There will be other pupils with conditions such as asthma or allergies that may require medication at school, so while not turning into a group of 'old women' chatting about various ailments, they can swap notes and be aware of the fact that they are not alone in having a medical condition.

How the Teachers May React

Most parents we talked to found teaching staff caring, sympathetic and willing to take on the extra responsibility. Many knew very little about diabetes and were anxious to learn as much as possible. Many requested a visit from a diabetes specialist nurse, others felt explanations from parents or literature (such as the BDA school pack) were enough to give them a good knowledge of the condition and how to look after the child.

As you may have guessed, there was a very small minority of teachers who gave the impression of being unwilling to take on any extra responsibility. 'I really cannot be expected to make sure James is having snacks when no one else in the class is . . . ' one parent was told. James's mother quite rightly felt uneasy about having her son involved with a teacher who had this attitude. A word with the headmaster resulted in James being moved to a parallel class; a disruption the child could have done without at this time in his life but there was no way he could have had the other teacher 'looking after' him.

The mother of five year old Georgina became annoyed when the school refused to take responsibility for her daughter during swimming lessons. 'I had to leave work and go to the swimming baths to supervise. Georgina's twin sister became very upset and resentful about the situation so, to keep the peace, I ended up going twice a week for two terms as they were in different classes. It was only when I threatened to take the twins away from the school that they relented and decided nothing drastic was going to happen as long as Georgina had her mini Mars bar first.'

One teacher insisted on calling another teacher away from lessons whenever nine year old Jenny felt hypo. This caused a disruption to both classes and Jenny felt uncomfortable and embarrassed. As her teacher was uneasy with the situation and life was becoming difficult for Jenny, her parents decided it was best to move her to another school in the area.

Luckily, these sort of incidents were very few and far between. Most parents found no problems in the teachers accepting their child back as diabetic and school life carried on as normal. Some even found themselves concerned by the over-confidence of staff in the early days of their child being diagnosed. Indeed, one mother actually became uneasy when her three year old's nursery school told her that they felt able to cope without her help right from the start.

'I offered to drop in once a day to make sure everything was going okay but they told me it wouldn't be necessary. They didn't seem to find any problem in having Alexander there and I spent weeks worrying about things. Of course, once I'd got over the nagging anxiety and wanting to be there all the time I was very grateful at how firm they had been with me. At first, though, I felt annoyed . . . as if I was being pushed out.'

One certainly can't blame Alexander's mum for being concerned over what she regarded as a rather 'laid-back' attitude. After all, he was very young. But she agrees it's vital to let go of your child, diabetes or not – and the sooner the better. A child will not thank you for trying to take away his independence or making him feel 'different'. There may be times when you have to appear at school for some reason connected with diabetes: as you will see later in this chapter, the clinic may ask you to check blood sugar levels before lunch at school. But if this happens at all it will only be very infrequently – maybe only three days running in a year. You must do it even if your child protests, but please do not feel compelled to make special journeys to do finger pricks 'just in case' your child's blood sugars might be high or low.

As long as you feel happy with the attitude of the staff at your child's school and feel that you have educated them the best way you can, leave well alone. However, if you find them negative or unhelpful in any way you must sort the problem out quickly. After all, a school which holds little store by pastoral care is surely not one you would wish your child to attend.

Yet however helpful everyone at school may be, there are often minor misunderstandings, all of which can be sorted out. These include:

School Dinners

There are various permutations of lunch which vary from school to school. Many schools offer a cafeteria-style choice which means there is bound to be something your child actually likes. But it also means that if he's too young (or unreliable) he may choose the wrong kinds of food. If you feel this is so, the lunchtime supervisor should be alerted and told how to encourage him to eat the right foods (including enough carbohydrate to see him through the afternoon) and steer him away from the wrong ones (the ultra-sweet syrup puddings). Try and instil sensible eating habits in your child, reminding him that by eating foods which may unnecessarily push up his blood sugars he is only cheating himself. You may well be surprised at how sensible he can be even at a very young age. Diabetic children quickly learn to recognise the needs of their own bodies.

If your child's school allows packed lunches the problem is virtually solved for you: just put whatever your child likes that is also right for him into the lunchbox. The only risk is that he will swap his high-fibre cereal bar for someone else's chocolate.

The biggest problem as far as school dinners are concerned is when there is a fixed menu with no choice and no option of a packed lunch. Many children complain about or simply don't eat their lunch at all. Most claim to detest the compulsory meal that is served up – often with just cause. One mother asked her child's headmaster whether he could make an exception and allow a packed lunch for her daughter who claimed she never touched a mouthful of the school lunch. The mother was given the curt reply: 'That would be a big problem. All the others would complain and find reasons why they should have a packed lunch and we simply cannot cope. She will just have to eat the lunch we provide.' Not wishing to make a fuss, which she would have had every right to do, or single her daughter out as 'different', the mother had a quiet word with the class teacher who saw to it that the child had a roll and an apple every day from the staff dining room. Not the perfect solution but at least the child had enough carbohydrate without suffering the embarrassment of a major fuss.

Sometimes there are misunderstandings if a child feels on the verge of a hypo and asks for the treacle tart to push up his blood sugars, only to be met with 'You're not allowed that, you're diabetic!' Whoever is on duty at lunchtime whether teacher, dinner lady or 'server' (usually an older pupil) should have an understanding of what diabetes is all about. They will have to trust that he is telling the truth – he probably will be.

Some mothers told us that their offspring were most upset and indignant when denied second helpings because they had diabetes. They claimed portions to be insufficient and needed more to curb their hunger. In this case, they should be treated no differently from other starving pupils! Most schools serve water at lunchtime so the question of drink does not arise. However, if your child's school serves squash make sure you provide a flask or small carton of low-calorie squash every day to stop him from drinking the ordinary variety.

Snacks

There are two possible dilemmas that may arise with snacks in school: *type* and/or *timing*.

If your child's school does not allow snacks to be brought in for break-time then you are going to have to explain to the headteacher that the child needs to eat something containing carbohydrate between meals. This could be a sandwich, banana, low-fat crisps or digestive biscuits. Biscuits are often a popular choice as a store can be left at school and eaten when required. Assuming the message that a diabetic child must eat carbohydrate between meals has got through, an exception will undoubtedly be made. If the school runs a tuck-shop you will have to hope you can trust your child not to buy a chocolate bar every day. Not giving him money rarely helps; children have crafty ways of smuggling their pocket money to school or collecting odd coins left around the house. Tipping off whoever runs the tuck-shop may be a good idea but hopefully your child's own conscience will help him to make the right decisions: fruit, plain or cheese biscuits and cereal bars are good choices.

Timing of snacks can be difficult if your child needs them at a different time to the scheduled breaks. A mid-morning snack works in fairly easily as break often falls smartly between breakfast and lunch (unless you have an unusually long car journey to school). An afternoon snack may be more awkward as there is often no break from lunch until going-home time. Older children, usually over eight, can train themselves into a routine and check their watch or classroom clock and discreetly eat their snack on time. Younger children will almost certainly have to be reminded and the teacher may be too busy to always remember. One inventive teacher appointed a special 'biscuit monitor' every week to make sure seven year old Suzy had her snack on time. Her classmates felt important when chosen for this responsible job (which certainly carried more kudos than handing out pencils!).

When Suzy was considered reliable enough to remember the snack herself, her classmates wanted to keep the job in an honorary capacity.

A watch with an alarm pre-set to go off at snack time is another idea so long as no one in class finds it off-putting!

Hypos at School

However good your child is at remembering snacks, there are bound to be times when his blood sugar level drops too low and he feels hypo. As you will have read in Chapter Three there is sometimes no real reason at all why a hypo occurs. This should not cause any concern as long as the hypo is treated in its early stages; before it becomes so advanced that the child actually becomes unconscious. Staff and fellow pupils must be made aware that, should your child complain of feeling dizzy, faint or have blurred vision, he must have immediate access to his supply of hypo-stoppers.

Most children – certainly those above the age of five – will usually recognise their early warning signs and, if the store of glucose is within easy reach, will be able to help themselves. But if they are away from wherever the supplies are kept the food should be brought to them by a member of staff or older child who can make sure they eat something sugary quickly and follow that up with something starchy (such as a biscuit) to stop the glucose levels falling again. It is not a good idea for a young child to wander off alone with a friend of his own age, as they could well dither around and become distracted, resulting in a full-blown hypo.

One mother said: 'Joseph told his teacher he needed some sugar and she sent him off alone to find his glucose tablets. Half an hour later he was found in the sickroom nearly unconscious. His box had been moved and he hadn't the strength to find someone to help.'

One seven year old was despatched to find a chocolate bar for her friend with diabetes. She came back empty-handed having eaten it!

It is important that you impress upon the staff how easy a hypo is to treat if caught early. The pale, listless pupil will be restored to his normal bouncing self within minutes. But if ignored, the situation could become serious and he may not be in any fit state to eat or drink. Should this unfortunate situation arise, he should not be made to swallow as this would be very dangerous, but a sugary solution such as Hypostop (see Chapter Three) must be rubbed into his gums.

Very young children may not be able to recognise signs of an impending hypo and their teacher should keep a look-out for a sudden change in behaviour. A pale, listless child with a faraway look in his eyes means action must be taken quickly. Naturally, teachers have a lot on their plate with many other children to watch over. But do ask that an extra eye is kept on yours.

Should you be summoned when your child has a hypo? Definitely 'yes' if it's serious and he has become unconscious. But in the experience of those parents we talked to, the chances of this happening are rare. Very few had been called upon to make the dramatic dash to school. Mild hypos may have happened but these had usually been successfully dealt with and forgotten.

It is worth asking your child (or teacher) to keep you informed of frequent signs of low blood sugars; this may mean his insulin dose is too high for the active life he leads at school. If months go by with no sign of hypos at school and there are high blood sugars when he comes home, he may not be having enough insulin. These are situations that may lead to your diabetes nurse asking you to go to the school to do pre-lunch tests (if the child is old enough he will be able to do his own).

Exercise

You will need to provide extra carbohydrate for your child to take before heavy exercise as the energy he uses may make his blood sugars drop too low. Most parents find chocolate mini bars most convenient (and the children won't refuse them!). How much carbohydrate your child needs depends on the amount of exercise he will be doing. A slow game of rounders may need nothing at all whereas an energetic country dancing session needs one mini bar at least. However, it is advisable to err on the safe side and give the extra snack. Exercise is covered in detail in Chapter Seven.

How Far Should You Become Involved?

Apart from making sure the teachers know enough about diabetes and checking that supplies of snacks and hypo-stoppers are topped up, your involvement with the school should be no more than it would normally be. If you are forever popping in or volunteering as a helper on school outings your child is going to get irritated and embarrassed. He may not want to be singled out or molly-coddled and children often find their parents embarrassing anyway.

A discreet word with the teacher every so often when you collect your child from school should be sufficient to let you know he is coping, and if there is anything you need to be told you will probably hear about it. Try and relax: you may not believe it, but plenty of children with diabetes go to boarding school and actually live through the experience!

It's a good idea for your child to carry a BDA identity card in his blazer or brief-case giving details of home and hospital phone numbers in case of emergency. If he has a necklace or bracelet saying that he has diabetes let the school know that you would like him to wear this even if there is a jewellery ban. But don't force him to wear it if he doesn't want to; he may see his ID bracelet as a symbol of 'being different'. Until your child is old enough to travel to and from school without an adult there is really no need for him to wear jewellery as identification to school.

School Outings

Day trips should not pose any worries provided the usual snacks and glucose tablets are taken along. Your child's teacher will know the times he needs his snacks and will no doubt make sure he eats them. Trips which involve staying away from home can also be undertaken providing the school are happy to take responsibility for overseeing injections and so on. It's unlikely a child who is too young to be doing his own injections would be going on a school trip that involved overnight stays; these usually come into a child's life when he is ten or older. But should the occasion arise when he is young, don't say 'no' unless you are absolutely sure it can't be done . . . there's every chance that it can. If your child is going on any kind of school trip then it is a good idea for him to wear identification just in case there is an accident.

School Supplies

A large packet of digestive biscuits, Lucozade (small bottles are easiest to manage), glucose tablets and a pack of mini chocolate bars should be sufficient for a few weeks. If you feel your child may need it, supply a bottle of Hypostop. A miniature jar of honey could substitute for Hypostop. Store biscuits in an airtight container to prevent them going soft, and put everything together in a plastic storage box (they come in all shapes, sizes and colours). Ask the teacher to keep supplies somewhere that is easily accessible for the child. The staffroom or first-aid cupboard might be suggested, but having to leave the classroom for a snack seems an unnecessary interruption. Check with your child or his teacher when you think supplies might be running low and be ready to replenish them when necessary.

Journeys To and From School

If you share a school run (that is, take turns with another parent or two to ferry the children to and from school) don't even consider giving it up or you will live to regret it! One mother told us of her experience: 'I arranged to take and collect Gemma every day myself for the first week that she was back at school. The idea was that the run I shared with a neighbour would revert to normal once I was happy that Gemma would not be hypo in the car. Although everything had been fine I still felt uneasy about someone else having to deal with any difficulties that might arise. I kept putting off sharing the run until my neighbour became fed-up with the situation and decided to share with someone else. After half a term I felt satisfied that Gemma would be fine and you've guessed what happened. It was too late . . . I couldn't find anyone else. A year later I'm still in the same boat . . .'

Don't assume that you are the only person capable of handing over the glucose tablets! School runs are invaluable and all you need to do is put the other mum in the picture and give her a supply of glucose.

Dilemmas sometimes occur if you do not allow snacks in the car and the other mother does. If the journey home is not the right time for your child's snack you probably won't want him to have the extra food – certainly not if it's chocolate. More than one mother found her child near to tears because his friends were allowed chocolate bars on the way home and he wasn't. But you cannot stop people carrying on with their own lives and your child has to learn the hard way.

Try having a word with your co-driver as most fellow mums are sympathetic to the feelings of children. Offer to supply something that your child can eat as well . . . if you really don't want him to eat at that time how about some sugar-free chewing gum? No harm will be done provided she doesn't deposit it all over the car!

Treats

If there's a birthday to celebrate in your child's class there may be cake or sweets on offer. Don't deny your child this pleasure and let the teacher know that the occasional celebratory treat will be fine. The chances are it will be handed out at breaktime anyway so he can run off the excess sugar in the playground.

Being Absent

Once your child has been diagnosed, treated and (if he was unwell) is feeling better, there is no reason why his attendance at school should be any different to that of a non-diabetes child. Obviously there will be occasional hospital visits but these can usually be arranged to coincide with school holidays. As far as actual illness goes, diabetes will not make your child more likely to suffer from other ailments or catch more infections. If he was below par before diabetes was diagnosed you will notice how much more robust he appears once he is on insulin. He will have far more energy and may recover from common colds more quickly than previously when his body was becoming more and more run-down.

If he is unlucky enough to have a bad bout of 'flu or a sickness virus you may find that his blood sugar levels are affected and you will have to monitor him carefully at home, giving extra insulin if necessary to stop the blood sugars rising so high that they produce ketones (see Chapter Nine). However, nearly all the mothers we talked to said that their children remained healthy. Only a very few had been particularly poorly and if this had been the case parents were usually able to stabilise them at home. Most children's blood sugars were unaffected by colds and minor infections.

In fact, people with diabetes in general seem to take little time off from school (or work). Perhaps subconsciously they are proving their point: that they are not 'different'.

Chapter 9

Special Situations

*'When Emma was diagnosed as having diabetes
I asked the doctor if I should cancel our summer
holiday. "What on earth for?" was all he said. Since
then we've been to Australia and the Far East . . .'*

*'Illness can be tricky . . . but if you know what
to expect you soon learn to cope . . .'*

*'Diabetes has not stopped Harry from doing
anything. He's probably been to more birthday
parties in the last year than ever before.
You learn how to be flexible . . .'*

Life Out of Routine

There are going to be occasions when your child's routine will have to change. Social events, holidays and a bad bout of illness may throw your guidelines (and your child's blood sugars) completely.

But as we've explained earlier, with experience and confidence you will be able to cope ably and, when necessary, bend your 'guidelines' to suit the circumstances. It may be hard to imagine this if you are only just learning about diabetes – but in the months to come you and your child will be your own experts!

Obviously you will seek the advice and back-up of your diabetes medical team when the need arises but you will find yourself able to organise most situations to suit everyone concerned.

Below is some information (including questions from our 'study group' which we have answered) that may help you to manage your child's diabetes in a variety of circumstances.

Holidays

Holidays are to be enjoyed and there is no reason why diabetes should put a stop to that! The world is your oyster: you can go anywhere you wish as long as you do some forward planning. None of the parents we spoke to had encountered any serious problems connected with diabetes.

Wherever you go, make sure your child is carrying some form of identification. It would certainly be a good idea for her to wear a necklace or bracelet. SOS Talisman and Medic-Alert are recognised around the world. If travelling abroad it is also a good idea to have an identification card written in the language of the country you are visiting. The BDA will be able to give you most of the information you will need.

For visits abroad, ensure your child has the appropriate vaccinations and any other medication she (and you) should be taking. Although vaccinations do not usually cause any special problems in people with diabetes you might find that your child's sugar levels rise and she may need some extra insulin to bring them back to normal.

If your child suffers from travel sickness, speak to your GP who will prescribe or recommend something to counteract this. If your child is sick, give her sweetened fruit juice about every hour to replace lost fluids and to replace the carbohydrate food she cannot tolerate. Even though she may vomit she will not develop ketosis because the sickness will cease when she stops travelling (blood tests will tell you how you are managing). If you are in a car you will be able to stop for breaks, but if you are travelling by some other form of long-distance transport you may need to give some extra quick-acting insulin to stop the blood sugars rising. Your doctor or diabetes nurse will suggest how much 'emergency' dose to give beforehand.

Rising sugar levels can also be caused by excitement. However, in this case there is no need to give extra insulin as sugar levels will return to normal when the child calms down. Try keeping to a normal routine for meals and snacks. If you make sure you carry extra biscuits, crisps or sandwiches there will be no need to panic if you are delayed or are unable to have your set meals on time.

Insulin and Travel

The best plan when travelling is to take double of everything: insulin, syringes, testing strips and lancets. If you use a pen, take a spare and double the amount of needles and cartridges. Take some disposable syringes as well. If the pen is lost or broken you can use a syringe to draw up insulin from the cartridge that normally goes in the pen. Practise drawing up insulin from the cartridge before you go away; don't try and put air into the cartridge before you draw up, or the rubber bung at the end will fly off and you will lose the insulin! It is a good idea to take a bottle of clear (quick-acting) insulin even if you don't already use it, just in case your child should become ill and require the extra insulin. Always carry this equipment in your hand luggage, along with whatever you use for blood-urine testing and hypostoppers. Do not let anyone take it away from you even for 'safe keeping' and make sure the bag is always within easy reach. If possible, someone else in your party should carry some of the 'duplicates' in case the precious bag gets lost or stolen. If two of you have the vital necessities you can feel at ease. Insulin should *not* be put in the hold of an aeroplane as it will freeze. It will be perfectly stable out of the fridge providing it is not placed in direct sunlight or in a warm place, such as the glove compartment of the car.

When travelling in warm weather, both in this country and abroad, keep insulin in a cooled vacuum flask or small cool-box. If there is no fridge available when you reach your destination you will have to keep the insulin in a bedside cabinet or under the bed. However, if you are holidaying in a very hot place you should make sure there is either a fridge at your disposal or a regular supply of ice for your flask or cool-box.

Keep Testing

Even though you are on holiday you cannot afford to stop blood or urine testing. In fact, you will probably have to test more frequently to gauge how your child is reacting to the difference in weather, activities and food.

These are some of the questions parents asked us about holidays.

Q Our nine year old son has recently been diagnosed as having diabetes and we are worried about the holiday we have booked. It's four months away but we still feel concerned. Should we cancel?

A Do not cancel your holiday! Your family will never forgive you and there is really no need to do so. It is understandable you are concerned as he has been recently diagnosed, but by the time you are set to go, diabetes will certainly seem easier to manage. You have plenty of time to plan your holiday, make lists of what you need and talk it through with your diabetes team. It may seem a big step now but you will be surprised at how quickly you and your child will adapt.

Q We have a long-haul flight to America ahead of us. The plane leaves at 10 am so we will have to get up at 6 am. Alex usually has his morning insulin at around 8 am. Can I give it to him earlier? Also, the flight lasts eight hours and the time difference is five hours (we are ahead of the US so the day will be longer). When should I give him his evening insulin? What about the return trip?

A Give Alex his normal insulin with breakfast at 6 am. He will require a snack about every two hours until his meal is served on the plane. Carry snacks with you in case a meal or the flight is delayed. As the day is five hours *longer* it may be as well to give an extra dose of quick-acting insulin before his tea-time meal on the plane (check the dose with your diabetes nurse). Then, unless a blood test shows his sugars to be very low, give the usual evening dose of insulin before supper when you have arrived in America. The day will be five hours *shorter* on the return trip. Give the usual insulin before supper on the day you leave and the next dose next 'morning', on the return trip as west-east flights are invariably overnight.

Q My children would love to go on a day trip to France. This involves a very early start and a late bedtime on our return. I'm also not sure when we will be able to eat during the day (and what!). Please help.

A You can either have breakfast early at home or *en route*, but check that they actually serve breakfast on the ferry before you go! Take snacks such as high-fibre bars or biscuits, and even some sandwiches in case of delays – but there are plenty of places to eat in the French ports. If you are going on an organised tour find out the times you are scheduled to stop for food. If you are visiting a hypermarket you will have the opportunity to buy food for the return journey. Give your child the usual insulin before the evening meal, wherever you decide to have it! This can be up to an hour or two before or after the normal supper time. But don't forget the evening snack, wherever you are, whether you are back home or still on the road.

Q When we are on holiday Ben does nothing but swim. What should I do about insulin, snacks etc.?

A This will require some blood tests. On the first day, give Ben the normal insulin dose and make sure he has a good breakfast containing long-lasting carbohydrate (see page 75). He will be using a lot of energy and hot weather can cause hypos. Let him eat ice-cream. Encourage him to drink fruit juice and eat high-fibre snacks such as cereal bars with his drinks. In the beginning check his blood sugar regularly, say four times a day. Explain how important this is. If you find his sugars are low or he has frequent hypos, reduce his pre-breakfast insulin. He may well not want to eat much if it is very hot but make sure he drinks plenty of sweetened fluids to stop him becoming dehydrated. After the first few days you will see a new pattern emerging to which you can adjust food and insulin.

Q Do all countries follow the same principles that we do for diabetes care? Would there be any kind of problem if we needed a doctor or emergency supplies?

A Most countries follow more or less the same principles. Finding a doctor abroad through your hotel or courier should not be a problem. However, before you travel check that your insurance covers your child with diabetes. If travelling to Europe complete form E111 from the DHSS. Some countries do not use U100 insulin (as we do), they use U40 which should only be drawn up in U40 syringes. A comparable insulin to the one your child uses should be available. The BDA produce travel leaflets covering many countries which will provide this type of information for you.

Q What special precautions should I take for my seven year old daughter when going abroad? Is there any extra equipment that I might need?

A Here's a list of everything you need to take abroad. It would be wise to take double of everything (see page 111):
- insulin
- syringes
- pen
- testing strips and lancets.

You will also need:
- log-book for blood/urine test results
- ketone-testing strips
- Glucagon and/or Hypostop
- ID jewellery and/or card
- glucose tablets, snacks, flask or cool-box
- form E111 from the DHSS if travelling inside EEC.

Oh, and don't forget the sun-tan lotion!

Q I've heard that airlines will provide a diabetic meal if you order it in advance. This sounds like a good idea. Should I do this?

A It is best *not* to order a diabetic meal for the plane, they usually contain little or no carbohydrate. Children's meals are usually a safe bet as they often include mashed or chipped potatoes which tend to go down well.

Q Will there be any problem going through customs with syringes etc.? I know how strict the airlines are and we don't want to be mistaken for drug addicts!

A Make sure you have identification. A letter from your hospital or GP stating that the child has diabetes may be helpful. It is also a good idea to have identification in the language of the country you are visiting. Here again, the BDA will have the relevant information.

Q Does hot weather affect diabetic control? I've heard that it can cause hypos. Is this why saunas are banned?

A Yes, hot weather can affect control. Warm skin can cause insulin to be absorbed quicker, which may lead to hypos. You may find your child needs to have her insulin nearer her meal as her blood sugars may be lower than usual. Saunas are *not* banned, but make sure your child always has a starchy snack first and does not take them alone. It's not a good idea for anybody to stay in a sauna or jacuzzi for long period of time. Ten to fifteen minutes is usually the recommended limit.

Q Tom usually has his supper at around 5 pm. On holiday we will be eating later, around 8 pm I expect. How do I fit injections into this new routine?

A Tom will need a snack instead of his usual meal at 5 pm; then there should be no problem having his injection, and then eating a full meal around 8 pm.

Christmas and Birthday Parties

These treats don't come often so why not turn a blind eye and let your child enjoy herself? Doctors agree that children with diabetes should be brought up as 'normal' and that includes enjoying treats. Don't feel annoyed if well-meaning but forgetful friends or relatives bring your child sweets when they visit. As we have already explained, these can be given after high-fibre meals, before exercise or as hypo-stoppers on 'ordinary' days. Don't suggest they bring 'Diabetic' chocolates next time they visit as they serve no valuable purpose and are an expensive waste of money.

Q Adam has been invited to a friend's party. This is the first time he will face plates of 'forbidden foods' since developing diabetes. Should we trust him to eat only sandwiches and crisps or would it be easier to make an excuse and not let him go?

A Do let Adam go to the party! He will never accept his diabetes if you stop him leading an active and normal life. He will certainly feel 'different' if he doesn't go. It will not matter if he has sweet party food. Just put it down to a boy enjoying himself. Although the odd high sugar won't do any harm, you may well find his blood sugar is actually low afterwards due to all the running around – so don't forget the bedtime snack.

Q What on earth does one do about injections for birthday party teas? My eight year old daughter can do her own injections but refuses to do this at a forthcoming party. Would it be a good idea if I arrived before tea and did the injection myself? The same question also applies to tea invitations straight from school.

A If your child cannot be persuaded to give her own insulin at the party then let her inject afterwards when she gets home. Just make sure she has a substantial snack to cover it, before bed. If *you* go to the party with her insulin this will almost certainly embarrass her.

Q My twelve year old daughter has been invited to a 'sleep-over' party. She will take her insulin with her but I'm not sure that she will remember to leave a twenty to thirty minute gap before supper. Would it be acceptable if she injected immediately before the meal? Also, I know the girls are planning a midnight feast . . . they are all taking something and I can imagine what will be consumed. What restraints should I put on Sally?

A The twenty to thirty minute gap is not imperative. It's better to inject immediately before the meal rather than to leave it any longer. At twelve, Sally will have a good idea what she should be eating. If she does consume sweet food, once again, the odd high sugar in the morning will not harm her. She should still have a bedtime snack. But don't rely on the midnight feast replacing this snack; if the food is sweet it will not be long-lasting enough carbohydrate to get her through the night.

Q All young children's birthday parties seem to end with a 'going home' bag containing the most sugary sweets imaginable and a piece of sickly birthday cake. Should I ask the birthday girl's mother not to put such things in my daughter's party bag or will this be embarrassing for all concerned?

A Let your daughter have her party bag. Give her the sweets or cake when she exercises or after a high-fibre meal. However, if she wants to eat some on the way home, that's fine – it's a treat, remember? It's as well to explain that she's being allowed to do this as it's a special occasion or she may think she can eat sweets ad lib.

Q What does one do about Christmas treats such as chocolate decorations on the tree and Advent calendars with a sweet a day? Is it best to stop this kind of thing altogether?

A A chocolate a day from the Christmas tree or Advent calendar will not do any harm as they are usually pretty small anyway. If you are still concerned, then give the chocolate after a meal or before exercise.

Out and About

Your child can go anywhere, do virtually anything as long as some thought is put into it. She should have access to glucose tablets at all times and carry identification, especially if you are not with her. Even the most convoluted schedules can have injections, snacks and meals fitted into them – really!

Q Where is the best place to give a child insulin when visiting a restaurant? Do other customers find it offensive? I know the obvious answer is the toilet but they are often very unhygienic.

A We understand your dilemma. Insulin pens make all this easier as you don't have to draw up the insulin. However, some people have no qualms about drawing up at the table. You can inject through clothes, so your child won't have to bare her body! One nine year old boy we know stands up and injects through his jeans into his bottom while still talking to his friends!

Q We have tickets for a late matinee at the theatre which would mean supper some hours after Jodi's usual injection time. I can make sure she eats snacks in the theatre but how much and what should she be eating bearing in mind that the morning insulin dose will be wearing off?

A Make sure Jodi has a snack at her normal supper time and again two hours later. This should be no problem in the theatre with chocolate, ice cream etc. circulating. Try and encourage her to eat something a little longer acting than just sweets: unsweetened popcorn is a good idea. Give the injection before the supper, *not* before the theatre (i.e. after the snacks).

Q My ten year old son desperately wants to go to Cub Camp. He does his own injections but I am afraid that he will forget and neglect his routine. Is it at all feasible for him to go?

A Speak to the people who will be looking after him at camp. It would be an idea if one person took on the responsibility of reminding him about his injections and snacks. Ensure all the adults know about diabetes and what it means. Explain your son's hypo symptoms and leave a contact number. Parents are always concerned when a child with diabetes is away for any length of time. But do let him go; he will more than likely cope admirably. Incidentally, an alarm watch (shock-proof and waterproof to cope with Cub activities!) would be of real benefit here, then he won't forget his snacks!

Q My son Joseph loves Indian food but whenever we go out for a meal he eats so much his blood sugars go sky high. I've heard that it is possible to give extra quick-acting insulin to cover an especially large meal. Is this possible?

A Yes, you can give an extra dose of quick-acting insulin, mixed in with his normal dose (see Chapter Three). Start with an extra one to two units then test an hour or so after the meal. If the tests are high then add another one to two units next time, depending on the results. If the blood sugar test result is under 10mmol/l, then you know you have got it right.

Illness, Stress and Minor Ailments

Because your child has diabetes does not mean she is any more likely to catch coughs, colds or childhood illnesses. However, if she does become unwell then particular care should be taken. This is because illness can cause a rise in blood sugar levels. Under *no* circumstances should insulin be stopped, even if your child is off her food. As you now know, if there is not enough insulin in the body, fat will be broken down to make energy resulting in the production of ketones, the build-up of which can eventually lead to coma.

Incidentally, ordinary medicines have only a minute sugar content so may be used, but there are many sugar-free alternatives available if you prefer.

What To Do

If your child is unwell, check her blood sugar levels regularly, at least two hourly and test the urine for ketones. If the sugar level is high and/or the urine shows ketones then your child will need extra insulin; she might need extra doses of quick-acting insulin. It's a good idea to contact your diabetes specialist nurse or doctor to find out how much extra to give, and when.

If your child is off her food, give her sugary drinks to maintain her carbohydrate intake. A glass of Lucozade or cola hourly should be sufficient, and further on in this chapter are some alternatives.

If your child vomits twice, or more, then contact your doctor or take her to the Accident and Emergency department of your nearest hospital as children can easily become dehydrated.

Suggested List Of Foods When Unwell

Each of the following contains 10g of carbohydrate:

Lucozade	50ml/2fl oz
Cola	100ml/4fl oz
Fruit juice	100ml/4fl oz
Milk	200ml/7fl oz
Ice-cream	50g/2oz
Yoghurt (half a pot)	50g/2oz
1 small banana	
1 pear, orange or apple	
Sugar or glucose	2 level teaspoons/2 lumps
Glucose tablets	3 tablets

Please don't imagine that every time your child catches a cold her sugar levels will rise. Many parents report no problems at all with the usual childhood ailments.

Hospitals and Illness

Q My three year old recently had a bad bout of measles and had to be given extra short-acting insulin to keep her blood sugars under control. She refused all solid foods and we felt that constant sugary drinks were doing more harm than good. Is there anything else we could have done?

A You seem to have done all the right things. Providing the blood sugar levels are controlled it is alright to give sugary drinks during periods of illness, when your child is off her food. See our list of other foods for further ideas. If you count exchanges (see page 81) don't worry too much that your child is not having the right amount but make sure she has small amounts, frequently.

Q My eight year old ended up in hospital due to a bout of flu and constant vomiting. She was very unhappy there and now at the first hint of a sniffle becomes frightened. What can we do to prevent this happening again?

A The best thing would be to start frequent blood testing at the first hint of a sniffle. If the sugar levels go up then increase the insulin and follow the guidelines at the beginning of this section. Make sure you know how much more insulin to give before your child becomes unwell again. Your diabetes specialist nurse will advise you. Act sooner rather than later, then your child need not be admitted to hospital so she will not feel frightened in future.

Q **Should I keep my son at home if he has a common cold? I'm anxious that things will escalate and feel he would be better off at home. I have kept him off school in the past although his blood sugars have stayed normal.**

A If your child's blood sugar levels are normal there is no need to keep him off school, unless he has a temperature. Try not to treat him any differently because he has diabetes – just take the normal care. Tell his teacher you are concerned and explain that if he is thirsty or leaving class to go to the toilet frequently, to let you know.

Q **My daughter's blood sugars sometimes go very high with no apparent cause. Can this mean she has some kind of virus or infection without showing any symptoms?**

A Sugar levels can go high for no real reason, although many causes have been explained throughout this book. It's unlikely she has had a virus or infection without showing symptoms. Look at the other reasons why this may have happened; has she missed an injection? Has she had a hypo? Has she eaten anything sugary that she hasn't told you about? If sugar levels are continuously high then she may be brewing an infection, but a one-off high sugar is not a cause for worry.

Q **My ten year old daughter's sugar levels go up whenever she has an exam, even if it's a simple test taken at Brownies. Is this normal and what should I do about it?**

A It is true that stress and worry can cause a rise in blood sugar levels. Children's exams are over fairly quickly so there would be no need to alter the insulin, unless your child worries continually for days before the event, causing her sugar levels to stay high over a period of time. Try to talk her worries through with her; reassurance may be all she needs. However, when she is older and her exams continue for weeks then her insulin may well need increasing to cope with the stress. Excitement can also cause blood sugars to rise.

Q I've heard people with diabetes are more prone to gum disease and tooth decay. Is this true?

A In people with well-controlled diabetes this is not the case. However, poorly controlled diabetes can lead to gum infections which in turn lead to tooth decay. Your child, like any other, should have regular dental check-ups.

Q My daughter would like to have her ears pierced. I have been told that this is not suitable for her as she would be likely to develop an infection. She is very upset and I wanted to have a second opinion.

A There is absolutely no reason why your daughter should not have her ears pierced provided it is done at a reputable beauty salon with sterile equipment. So long as she does not 'fiddle' with her ears or remove the sleepers for the recommended six weeks she is no more likely to have infection than anyone else.

Q My son has a verruca. I bought some ointment which says 'not suitable for people with diabetes'. Why is this and what should I do about the verruca?

A The ointment probably contains acid which would not be appropriate for older people with diabetes who may have nerve damage to the feet. As for verrucas, it's best to leave them alone to clear up by themselves unless they are causing discomfort (wear a verruca sock when swimming). But, if necessary, see a state registered chiropodist who will be able to treat it. Foot care in people with diabetes is essential in case of nerve damage (neuropathy) in later life. It's never too early to start looking after the feet.

Chapter 10

Emotionally Speaking

*'I felt depressed for some months after the diagnosis.
Adam coped very well and always seemed cheerful.
In the end that's what got me out of it. It dawned on
me that he was the one with diabetes and if he was
okay about it, why shouldn't I be? . . .'*

*'The arguments in our house increased considerably.
My other daughter became very insecure and moody . . .'*

*'All my children have the same snacks at the
same time. That way, nobody can be singled out
as "lucky" or "different" . . .'*

Facing Diabetes as a Family

Some families find that they need outside help to enable them to
cope with the emotional impact of their child's diabetes. Their
doctor, diabetes nurse or GP will try to sort things out but if they
feel it necessary, they may suggest seeing a psychologist or
someone who is trained as a counsellor for such situations. Indeed,
many parents we talked to had been to a psychologist at some time
or another and most of them admitted finding it beneficial. Parents
who had not been for counselling were confident they could keep
problems under control within the family. Some even wondered
whether having professional help might sow the seeds of problems
where none had existed in the first place.

However, everyone agreed that talking helped greatly to relieve
pressures they felt. Whether this involved partners, friends, local
support groups or professionals the need to discuss feelings and
anxieties was obvious.

'I knew of someone who had a child with diabetes and decided to get in touch with her. The relief was enormous,' said one parent. 'Just hearing that, three years on, her son was healthy and leading a normal life was my therapy.'

Another told us: 'My husband had a client who had had diabetes for twenty years. Although they had not seen each other for some time I urged my husband to contact him. This man was so helpful and encouraging. He came over to show us the living proof that it was possible to be successful, healthy, good-looking – and have diabetes!'

Many parents agree that coming to terms with emotions and trying to accept the situation is far harder than getting to grips with the treatment. As for the 'patients', young children tend to accept whatever life throws at them far more readily than older children and adults. Adolescents are often particularly angry and unwilling to accept their diabetes. Not only do they have the turmoil of a changing body, they must also cope with adjusting to diabetes. The combination is likely to be explosive and needs particularly sensitive handling.

First Feelings

When told their child has diabetes some parents react almost as if the child had died. Great sadness, disorientation, insomnia, overwhelming preoccupation with the child and even anger are emotions frequently described. Sometimes talking about diabetes is a burden . . . yet it cannot be pushed to the back of one's mind. It is always there to worry about and question: 'Why my child? Why our family?' There may be a feeling of disbelief that there is no actual cure, or the hope that the doctors have made a mistake.

'Learning that Tom had diabetes made the whole family seem vulnerable,' explained one mother. 'We had jogged along for years thinking this kind of thing only ever happened to others. Now we were included. It was like a club I didn't want to join.'

It is only natural to grieve for the once perfect health of a child and this is encouraged by psychologists. But this period of mourning will end and you must face up to your child's diabetes. Once you can see that life goes on as normal you are well on the way to accepting the situation.

The strain on relationships between partners can be enormous especially if things were rocky before diabetes came along.

'Our marriage had not been right for some years and I think that Gemma's diabetes was a catalyst for the break-up. My husband argued with me over everything: Gemma's diet, her blood tests, her lifestyle . . . it was almost as if he was enjoying a new excuse for conflict.'

'I have a second cousin who has diabetes and my wife took out her anger on me from the beginning. The fault was all mine; my side of the family had given this to Simon . . .'

'My husband supported me when it first happened. He was fantastic. But once it became a part of our lives he lost interest. It's not that he doesn't care, it is simply that the responsibility is now mine. On reflection, I guess that means life is back to normal. He treats the diabetes as yet another domestic duty along with the cooking and housework!'

Sibling Demands

Brothers and sisters often resent the spotlight that is suddenly thrust upon the child with diabetes. Why is everyone fussing? Why does he get the extra presents? Why must we rush home for his injections? Why is so much thought put into her food and why can't I have an extra chocolate bar? Siblings who have previously had no axe to grind suddenly find one. Those who have always felt their brother or sister was the favourite have more fuel to add to the fire. Sometimes they fear they will be pushed to one side or not loved as much and sadly these fears sometimes go unrecognised. The consequence in one such case was disastrous.

'My thirteen year old daughter became ill with the slimming disease *anorexia*. She was in hospital for months and we were told it was her way of getting our attention.'

There can never be a right or wrong way to handle such delicate situations as so much depends on the individual concerned. But keeping things as normal as possible and playing down the diabetes goes a long way to help maintain the balance among siblings.

'I have tried to treat Sarah exactly the same as her brother, who does not have diabetes, right from the start. She was told off for the same things, given attention only when necessary and encouraged to do as much as possible for herself with a minimum of fuss. She is just five now and has had to grow up very quickly – too quickly perhaps – but that seems a small price to pay.'

Some parents found the refusal of the child without diabetes to co-operate with new eating habits a problem.

'I automatically switched to a diet that would be suitable for my daughter but her ten year old brother David would not accept this. He always complained, especially about the diet drink, and I gave in. I now buy diet *and* regular of everything. It's annoying but it works. To him, drinking diet Coke represented a change in *his* life, which he felt was unfair as he did not even have diabetes.'

If diabetes does not directly affect their lives, siblings are far less likely to have problems than if it is rammed down their throats. Again, the situation can be compared to having a new baby in the house with the attention, the demands, the anxieties and most of all the fear that they will now be second best. It is also important to reassure them that their brother or sister with diabetes will be healthy and is not going to be an invalid.

Hannah, an eleven year old, told us: 'I felt very worried at first because I thought Suzy was going to die. I imagined that she would be in hospital all the time and be really ill. When Mummy explained exactly what diabetes was and that Suzy would be fine, I stopped worrying and everything carried on as before.'

Eight year old Sam became very clinging and would not let his mother out of his sight. 'I thought that diabetes was catching and I would get it too,' he said. 'I kept dreaming that my brother was going to die, and then I would wet the bed. The doctor explained lots of things to me and I felt better. I stopped wetting the bed, too.'

Try and involve brothers and sisters as much as possible. Everything must be explained in some depth so that they do not feel excluded and are able to understand what is going on, and why.

Many parents have found counselling particularly helpful in removing the doubts and fears of siblings who often will not talk openly about their feelings. 'Someone trained to help can really get through to them,' explained one parent. 'Psychologists have the patience and the training to understand and put things right in a way that we are often unable to do.' A recent medical journal made a study of siblings of children with diabetes and reported a significant number felt that their families had become *closer* because of the diabetes. Surely this goes to prove that problems can be sorted out with patience and understanding?

If you had previously banned between-meal snacks in your household, the rules will have to change now to keep the peace. If the child with diabetes is the only one allowed a mid-morning biscuit there is bound to be trouble. Let his brothers and sisters join in and think of it as a treat – at least that's something positive for *them*. You should probably draw the line at handing out hypo-stoppers to the entire family; explain that these are a kind of medicine and they can have their own sweets and fizzy drinks at other times.

Diabetes as a Weapon

There are many ways in which children can use their diabetes as a weapon to draw attention to themselves. Refusing to do injections, refusing to eat, not co-operating with medical staff, letting hypos get out of control . . . they have the power to cause you continual worry. Yet none of this need happen and these kinds of problems can usually be solved before they get out of hand.

For instance, how should you react the first time your child refuses to have his injection? If he is very young then reasoning will have no effect simply because he will not be able to understand the implications of letting his blood sugars run high. In this case you will probably have to hold him in a firm grasp and push the needle in. Parents who have had to resort to force find it distressing at first but once the child gets used to the idea that the injection is going to be done *no matter what*, he realises it's easier to give in and get on with it.

If your child knows exactly why he must have his injections but refuses to do his own, or let you do them, try not to get angry. Don't beg either. If you show your anxiety he will have you exactly where he wants you. Every child knows how to wind up those closest to them and yours can certainly have you over a barrel with this one! Don't ever consider bribing. You could find yourself the victim of blackmail for years to come . . .

Keep calm. Try using your most matter-of-fact voice and say something like: 'All right, please yourself. You know very well that the injections are to keep you healthy. You could well end up in hospital and are going to look pretty stupid when the doctor asks what's gone wrong. Just remember, it's your diabetes and you are the one who must take care of it.'

Walk away, start doing something else. In most cases, better judgement will overcome your child and he will grudgingly get on with the injection. Screaming threats or begging will only show him what an explosive weapon he has. If you appeal to his integrity and put the ball in his court he will begin to realise that looking after his health is no one's responsibility but his own. You are not his keeper, and you trust him enough to look after his own life.

If problems continue, try talking about the situation. Explain again why he must have his injection and that before insulin was invented children became very ill and could not do all the things he can do. That little pin-prick is his life-line. Is diabetes really so bad? If nothing seems to work, then you are almost certainly going to need professional help. Speak to your doctor or diabetes specialist nurse and if they cannot help they will arrange for a psychologist to speak to your child and find out what's *really* bothering him. One way or another, things are bound to work out.

The same plan of action goes for refusals to eat. Even babies are capable of getting parents into a state over food. They can sense from a very young age how you will react, and treat mealtimes accordingly. When a baby won't eat it is important to keep your emotions under control. The baby with diabetes must eat, of course, to cover the insulin, but he will be too young to recognise that not eating brings on hypos. If your baby refuses his food, give him an alternative . . . something he will eat but nothing he likes so much that he'll for ever be refusing your first choice. It is tricky, but he will grow out of this difficult phase. Nearly all babies create havoc over food at some time or another but if you don't make a big fuss about it they soon give up.

Children who refuse to eat will soon realise that hypos are not very pleasant and can be prevented. Again, keep calm while explaining the facts. Parents often find that older children are worried about putting on weight and want to diet. This usually happens when they are teenagers and it is not to be dismissed lightly as it could lead to secret slimming. It is perfectly reasonable that your child wants to look good. Discuss this with your child's doctor and dietitian: they will be able to work out a suitable scheme of cutting down food and insulin accordingly so that it will not affect blood sugar control.

Attention Seeking with Hypos

One mother told us a hair-raising story of her teenage son who seemed to enjoy ending up in hospital after mega-hypos which often involved drinking, missing meals and having fits.

'Tom was at boarding school when he was found to have diabetes. Both my husband and I wanted him to come home and go to day school. Tom – then twelve – pleaded with us to let him stay where he was happy. However, about three years later things became very bad and virtually every week we were having to drive miles because Tom had been found unconscious at school. We were frantic with worry, but after a while it dawned on us that he seemed to revel in our visits at the hospital. The next time it happened we didn't go to see Tom in hospital. We phoned him and said that all this dashing backwards and forwards was not on. What was *really* bothering him?

'Eventually he told us that boarding was not turning out as he had hoped (nothing to do with his diabetes) and he wanted to come home. He had felt too embarrassed to admit it. This was his way of making us find out.'

Teenage problems are especially difficult to deal with: when a child reaches adolescence, communication seems to disappear completely for several years. This, too, is a delicate time when a child will want to know 'Why me? What have I done to deserve this?'

One father, with diabeteshimself, became riddled with guilt as arguments with his teenage son always culminated in: 'It's your fault that I have diabetes. Why did you have me in the first place?' But it's worth remembering that if your adolescent child didn't have diabetes to throw back in your face it would only be something else: 'Why am I so fat/spotty/ugly/skinny . . .' The teenage years are extremely hard work in the majority of households. See Chapter Eleven for more information about the teenage years.

Bingeing on Forbidden Foods

Anyone who has ever been on a diet will recognise the allure of forbidden foods. Many parents have told us they have discovered their child has been 'pigging' himself on chocolate. Everyone feels like a good binge sometimes and perhaps it is wise to turn a blind eye (very occasionally) and let your child get whatever craving he has out of his system.

There may sometimes be a more serious underlying cause. He might tell you that he binges, and then feels guilty, but doesn't know why he does it. If so, seek professional help immediately. There are all kinds of reasons for this behaviour which most parents are not equipped to fathom out.

In all cases of emotional conflict your biggest ally is support from others. Never let yourself or your child bottle up anger, guilt, worry or depression. Seek help from those you trust and admire. Almost every problem can be sorted out in the end with good advice and understanding.

When to Let Go

It is important that you make it clear to your child right from the start that it is his diabetes, not yours. He is the person who must ultimately become responsible for his treatment and his own actions. Once he realises this he is well on the way to becoming independent of you.

By the time they start secondary school the majority of children with diabetes will be capable of drawing up insulin and doing their own injections, interpreting blood test results and acting accordingly (with some advice from you and the medical team). By this time, too, your child will be wanting to go out with his friends unencumbered by adults. He will be able to do so if he can be trusted to act responsibly and in a mature way. If you have a child who is 'young' for his age you would probably not be happy to give him so much freedom in any case. All children are different and learn to do things at different times. Ask your child to teach a friend diabetes care, just as the doctor taught him. You will soon see how competent your child is. Go slowly and never put pressure on to 'take over your own diabetes'. He will do so when he's ready.

Chapter 11

Diabetes in the Teens

*'Sally was so easy before she reached adolescence.
When she was twelve she totally rejected her diabetes –
and everything else for that matter. Now, nine years
later she has sorted herself out and is a reasonable
human being again . . .'*

*'Tom always used his diabetes as an excuse for why he
couldn't fit into certain situations. Once he found a girlfriend
and had a steady relationship he stopped using
it as a security blanket and got on with life . . .'*

*'Teenagers are so ghastly.
Diabetes just gives them another reason to be so . . .'*

A Changing Child

Although this book is mainly concerned with children up to the age of twelve, one big question in your mind is bound to be: 'What happens when they are teenagers?' It might help to look ahead, into the teens, to get an idea of how diabetes can affect your child later.

All parents view the imminent arrival of their children's teenage years with apprehension: and with some justification! Even without a child having diabetes, the teens present fairly harrowing challenges to both child and parents.

A child developing diabetes during puberty is particularly hard: being faced with the traumas of a changing body as well as learning to cope with diabetes is enough to send the most level-headed of youngsters into a total spin. For the child who has had diabetes for some time, becoming a teenager means finally facing up to the demands that the condition entails. Whereas until then she has been able to leave it to her parents to worry about details of diet, insulin and so on, she now finds that she has to learn to take full responsibility herself and this really brings home the full implications of the diagnosis.

'Jenny had been exceptionally easy about her diabetes until she reached twelve,' said one mother. 'Suddenly she didn't want to know. She rejected our help and it took a couple of years for life to settle down. We found the hospital psychologist invaluable.'

Not all teenagers find it easy to adjust to this extra responsibility and perhaps it's not surprising that some totally reject the self-discipline which is needed. But surely it would be a rare and perhaps a worrying teenager, who did not go through at least a period of rebellion – in this case against diabetes?

The extent to which your child comes through the teens as a well-adjusted, level-headed young adult depends – as with all the other aspects of adolescence – on the love, support and understanding which she receives from friends, medical advisors and, above all, from the family.

The Growth Factor

The big feature of puberty is the sudden and dramatic increase in the secretion of sex hormones. Coupled with the more obvious bodily changes which this causes, it also results in an equally dramatic increase in the secretion of growth hormone, resulting in a major growth spurt. In girls this growth spurt occurs right at the beginning of puberty (which can start as early as ten), whereas in boys it does not occur until about two years later.

But growth hormone does more than just make you grow. It is a hormone which affects the *metabolism* and thus tends to raise blood glucose levels considerably. Normally the pancreas is able to compensate for this by secreting more insulin, so that children in puberty have much more insulin in their circulation than younger children. But in pubescents with diabetes, the pancreas is unable to respond in this way and a big increase in the dose of insulin is usually needed to compensate for the effects of increased growth hormone secretion.

Growth hormone is actually secreted in bursts rather than as a continuous trickle. A graph of growth hormone levels in the blood throughout the day looks like a map of the Himalayas! As a result, blood glucose levels in teenagers with diabetes are far more unstable than at other times of life. What's more, since the peaks of growth hormone in puberty are largely unpredictable, it is not possible to fine-tune diabetic control by adjusting insulin doses to the same extent as at other times of life.

Girls and their Periods

Where puberty in boys is fairly straightforward, girls have periods to cope with. The levels of oestrogens, the female hormones in the blood, go up and down at different times of the month. In most girls, changes in blood sugar levels at different times of the month are not enough to cause major problems, but it's surprising that more girls do not have greater problems with their diabetic control than they actually do.

However, in a small number of girls, blood sugars go haywire around period time, and the odd thing is that it seems to affect different girls in different ways. Many girls notice a sharp increase in their appetite during the week before a period, and this may lead to high blood sugars. Yet with experience and some finger-prick tests, they soon learn to increase the insulin dose at this time (and to reduce it as soon as the period arrives, of course).

Other girls, though, find that in the week or so before period time their sugar levels are low despite a huge appetite. Doctors do not really understand why this happens but the same thing seems to happen every month to the same individual. In this case, the insulin dose will have to be lowered to prevent endless hypos in the days before a period starts, and then increased again once the period has arrived.

Growing Appetites

Teenagers always seem to be hungry. Their appetite increases dramatically when they reach puberty and this is probably due to the increased levels of growth hormone and insulin. While ravenous hunger is a perfectly normal part of puberty (and probably necessary for all the growing) it can certainly complicate blood sugar control.

As you now know, the key to keeping blood sugars normal is balancing insulin to meals and exercise. In as far as meals are concerned, teenagers must make an attempt to relate the timing and doses of injections, not only to the size of their meals, but also to what they are eating, and how often.

The general idea is the same as at other ages, but problems may be exaggerated both by the size of the portions and by the unpredictability of meal-times, as the teenager becomes more and more independent and goes her own way. An insulin pen (see Chapter Three) often solves many of the problems simply because the child can inject quick-acting insulin to cover meals at the times she wishes to have them. This means one or two extra injections, but actually gives far greater flexibility. She can adjust the dose to what she is going to be eating and allow for any exercise later on. Some teenagers are reluctant to do this, but if they can be persuaded to give the idea a try they usually realise that it's far more practical for their hectic lifestyle and the regime takes them comfortably into adulthood where they may meet the demands of a job with less regular meal-times, bedtimes and so on.

'Tom took to the pen straight away,' said his father. 'He liked the look of it; getting away from syringes meant a great deal to him. He shows it to people quite matter-of-factly and now he's at university he finds it quite easy to fit in with the eating habits of other students. He injects himself through his clothes so expertly, no-one ever notices what's going on.'

Unfortunately, the facts are that the teenager's usual habit of eating snacks and junk food will not help blood sugar control, but it's the child herself who has to come to terms with this. There is simply no point in trying to prevent your child from enjoying a normal social life and there is every chance that you would make matters worse if you constantly nagged about her diet.

Weight Problems

Puberty results in a big dramatic change in size and shape. Everyone knows how teenagers – especially girls – can be painfully self-conscious. Every week there's a fresh surprise in the mirror, and the child is not always entirely happy with what she sees. Sometimes, this becomes an obsession to the point where it is out of all proportion and may lead to overeating or semi-starvation.

The presence of diabetes can add an extra dimension to these problems. Insulin tends to increase the appetite and the child might realise that keeping good blood sugars is actually making her put on weight. Consistently high blood sugars will lead to weight loss and if she realises this she may be tempted to drop her insulin (making her less hungry), run her blood sugars high, and lose weight.

Adolescence is a time for experimenting and rebellion but as with many experiments, they can soon turn into habits which in turn can become dangerous. Leaving off insulin injections altogether usually results in ketosis and possibly coma (as you know from when your child was first diagnosed) (see page 13).

Any parents of teenagers will tell you just how secretive their offsprings' behaviour can be and as often as not parents of a teenager with diabetes may have little idea that there are any problems. The first clue may be a difference between the child's own blood sugar results and the HbA_1 or Fructosamine levels that we talked about in Chapter Four. Any hint of eating disorders or your child letting her blood sugars run out of control deliberately should send you for specialist help.

Learning from Others

We have already mentioned the benefits of children spending time at BDA summer camps and if you can persuade an albeit reluctant teenager to go they will really benefit. Older children tend to discuss mutual problems with their peers and they can ask all those questions that they had been afraid to ask without feeling silly. They will probably learn more about their own condition than they have done in the whole of the previous year and discover that they are not the only ones with diabetes. It will soon dawn upon them that they *can* cope.

Rebels with a Cause

Adolescence is a time for rebelliousness. It is the stage when the child can, for the last time, see what she can get away with and where the limits are. This will include everything from staying out late at night to a surreptitious first cigarette (*smoking is a definite no-no for people with diabetes*) and the child's attitude to such things will have much to do with the parents' reaction.

'Drinking is a real worry,' one mother told us. 'You can't stop them going out with friends and as alcohol lowers the blood sugar there is always a risk of hypos. I've tried to instil in Robert that he should always eat plenty before he drinks and make sure he has starchy carbohydrate. He does eat sensibly but I worry whenever he's out late.'

It's not only the child who can use diabetes as a weapon either. The parent can turn it to advantage as well. For instance, if you were unhappy about the home influences of your child's friend you could try to stop your child going there by saying: 'You can't go to so-and-so's party because you won't be able to eat the food.' This is a very damaging thing to do; you are throwing the diabetes back at the child and using it for your own ends. The child will doubtless counteract by saying 'If you don't let me go, I won't take my insulin.' And who can blame her?

But more often than not, the conflict is far more subtle than this kind of example and does not lead to an argument. As with so many other things in adolescence, it is merely the child exploring how far the goal-posts can be moved and you should take the opportunity to talk things over with your child, discussing your own attitudes and beliefs. Your child can then examine them and form her own attitude to her diabetes.

It's important to understand that children are frightened by their diabetes. They need reassurance from you that they can cope with it. It's just that sometimes they have rather strange ways of asking for help!

How Good can Control Be in the Teens?

Every parent of a child with diabetes is going to worry about the possible long-term consequences for her health. But how far should you drive yourself crazy trying to achieve good control in adolescence when diabetes becomes more than usually difficult?

Complications of diabetes are virtually unheard of before puberty, and rare in the teens. The difficulty, of course, is that some problems may develop over many years. But does it make any difference to the risk in future years if the diabetes has been poorly controlled in childhood? Doctors' attitudes to diabetes management in the teens are changing nowadays because evidence suggests that the first few years of diabetes are the important ones as far as future complications are concerned.

Until recently many doctors have taken the attitude that the most important thing is to keep the child out of hospital, make sure she feels well, avoid hypos at all costs and make sure she enjoys a full life. Now it is possible to keep control of blood sugars at home by easy testing, coupled with hospital tests, doctors have become more aware of just how badly controlled most teenagers' diabetes is.

The fact is that the difficulty of obtaining good control should *not* put you off trying. But you have to realise that really good control is just not possible in most teenagers. If a child never has even a mild hypo, her blood sugars must be permanently too high and there is almost certainly scope for improvement in her diabetic control. If, on the other hand, she does experience minor hypos, but only if she is late with a meal, or has taken more exercise than normal, she is on the right track and appears to have her insulin, food and exercise well balanced. However, watching out for hypos is no substitute for testing. No-one wants their child having hypos all the time but to a minor extent these can be used as a yardstick if the child is not producing many finger-prick results.

It is equally important that a conscientious teenager does not feel it is her fault that her diabetes is not better controlled. Often, the extent to which one can try for better control has more to do with the child's personality than with the diabetes itself. With every child there must be a point where the diabetes is as well controlled as it can be without interfering with the child's lifestyle more than is absolutely necessary.

Remember, though, that the adolescent years do not last for ever and many a parent of a rebellious, difficult teenager – with diabetes or not – will testify that their child has come out of the experience the other end a responsible, caring, sensible adult.

Chapter 12

Diabetes in Babies

'My baby Sam was diagnosed diabetic not long after being born. Having to stick a needle in my tiny baby nearly killed me. It took almost a year to accept the horrible thing I had to do. But Sam is now five. He's healthy, clever and virtually injects himself. To him, it's a way of life and he thinks his friends who don't have to inject are the odd ones...'

'Alexander actually disliked having his nappy changed more than the injections...'

'I would say the problems one has with a young baby are magnified a hundred times if it has diabetes. But once you learn to cope, believe me, you can cope with anything...'

A Difficult Diagnosis

Although diabetes is becoming far more common in children it is still quite rare in babies. The thought of a tiny, helpless infant being used as a pincushion is most new parents' nightmare. The diagnosis in a baby is very difficult for the doctor to make, largely because the early signs, of going to the toilet frequently, or asking for drinks, are completely masked; you can't possibly know how many times the baby has wet his nappy, and crying with thirst could be mistaken for all sorts of other reasons. Very often the baby ends up in hospital with an infection which precipitates the knowledge that he does, in fact, have diabetes. By this time, he is often very ill with ketosis and dehydration.

Whatever the reason, if a baby has diabetes there is no way out of the normal treatment: balancing insulin with food and exercise however daunting this may seem. But parents cope – they have to.

'It's like being struck by lightning,' said one mother whose baby was three months old when diagnosed. 'You are so frightened, so desperately worried about this tiny human being. The biggest anxiety is that it cannot communicate at all. Everything is done by guesswork. But you would be surprised at how good you get at guessing and finding the right signs.'

Handling Your Baby

Having to inflict pain on your baby by pushing a needle into him is a horrifying thought but you must never be tempted to leave an injection out because you feel so bad about doing it. With plenty of love, cuddles and happy surroundings your baby will grow up accepting his lot in life without any presumptions that you are deliberately trying to hurt him. He will never have known life without injections and his day will include them along with other regimes that he will be learning. Your baby will probably find teething far more of an upset than injections.

The obvious problems with a baby who has diabetes are:
- feeding habits
- spotting hypo signs
- injecting
- testing for glucose.

The injections are probably the easiest part as you can have everything ready and inject while he's on your lap or on the changing mat waiting for a nappy change. Blood and urine testing can be more difficult but there are ways round each situation.

Injecting a wriggling baby may need expert help to start with and it is important to have the support of your diabetes nurse or a visiting community nurse right from the start. Any family members who are willing to make silly noises or faces to distract the baby's attention are invaluable. However, you'll soon learn how to hold your baby, distract him and inject expertly yourself . . .

Always give lots of cuddles afterwards to help him forget any slight pain. Remember though, an injection done swiftly feels like a gnat-bite . . . and the sensation does not linger for more than a few seconds.

As we explained in Chapter Three, you must rotate the injection sites to stop any lumps forming or altering the action of the insulin. The best places to inject a baby are the bottom and upper legs where there is most fatty tissue. Arms at this age are rarely chubby enough and are usually waving around in any case.

Testing Your Baby for Sugar

Urine testing can be done several ways and may be fairly hit and miss, literally! In fact, young babies often produce a stream on reflex when you are in the middle of changing their nappy, as all parents know to their cost! Have a cup handy at changing time to catch a possible specimen, or cup your hand over a boy's penis. Have glucose testing sticks at the ready and dip.

Terry towelling nappies can be squeezed into a small pot or onto the testing strip but there is a problem of washing powder or fabric conditioner altering the test result. This can be solved by putting a strip of cotton wool or a liner inside the nappy and then squeezing that out. Disposable nappies seem to be used more widely than terries these days and parents are often taught to place the urine stick in the wet pad, fold it over and squeeze really hard, as if wringing out a towel. This should provide enough urine to coat the test area.

An old-fashioned way of potty training was to put young babies, virtually as soon as they could sit unaided, onto the pot in the hope of catching everything possible. This is now discouraged normally, but might help in the case of urine testing, you might have an early potty-trained baby into the bargain! Remember to rinse the potty well after washing as cleansing preparations can affect the test result.

Another difficulty with urine-testing babies is that they tend to show sugar in the urine even if the blood glucose is only slightly above 10mmol/l so you need test sticks which read from 0–5% to give you a more accurate result. Regular ketone testing is also valuable. Babies are more likely to have ketones in their urine than older people. They burn up their fat stores far more readily, especially overnight when less insulin is circulating in the body, hence the appearance of ketones in the early morning urine test. Do not worry when ketones appear and disappear occasionally with no apparent cause but do speak to your doctor or diabetes nurse if you feel there is reason for concern.

The aim is for your baby to have as many sugar-free urine tests as possible. Your diabetes nurse will advise you on how many tests you should do and how to respond to the results.

Blood testing will, of course, give you a far better up-to-the-minute picture of what's going on and it's surprising how tolerant babies and young children can be of all the pricking required. Granted, it's not going to be easy to prick-test a wriggling tiny body but there's inevitably a way that, with practice, you will be able to perfect.

Because of the size and incessant clenching and clawing of tiny fingers, ear-lobes and heels often provide more successful test sites. Squeezing the sample onto the strip is going to be tricky but is by no means impossible. There are also devices to help: your diabetes nurse may provide you with a tube which 'sucks' the blood up and drops it onto the strip so that the sample lands accurately.

There are no hard and fast rules about which method of testing – blood or urine – you should use for your baby. Often a combination of the two will give an overall picture of how things are going. Your diabetes nurse is the best person to advise you on a plan of action.

How Do You Spot Hypos in a Baby?

This may well be your biggest worry, but it's not insurmountable. You will soon learn to understand your baby's hypo signs without him actually being able to tell you how he feels. Of course, babies cannot display the tell-tale signs of older children. They are not naughty as such, do not complain of a tummy-ache or look 'wobbly'. However, they often go extremely pale – translucent is how one mother described it – with a vacant expression. They may also become irritable and grizzly, sweaty or limp. If the hypo is progressing the limbs may twitch and jerk. The baby may even vomit.

Try to quickly think through a few points: is this the time the clear or cloudy insulin will be acting most strongly (see Chapter Three)? Has the baby had his regular amount of carbohydrate? Has he been more active than usual in the past twelve hours? Is this happening just before a meal when he needs more carbohydrate? A blood test can confirm a hypo and then you can act. A recommended hypo-stopper for babies is two fluid ounces of milk with sugar. Honey, jam or Hypostop squeezed onto the gums should also work. If things get really bad and you cannot get anything into the baby's mouth, you will have to inject Glucagon (as described in Chapter Three). If the baby is old enough to chew you can give sugary biscuits or glucose sweets.

You really have to 'think on your feet' in order to spot hypos in babies, but given time and experience this will become second nature. As one father told us proudly: 'We were so used to watching and acting on Adam's hypos signs that we were completely taken aback when he turned round one day and said "I feel shaky". I think he was about two years old. That was a real turning point – after that we could more or less rely on Adam to tell us himself. His usual expression was: "Get the sweets daddy", but at least we knew that he was able to recognise his own symptoms.'

Feeding Your Baby

You may be wondering whether a very young baby who is not yet on solids can possibly get enough carbohydrate from milk feeds alone. In fact, both breast and bottled milk contain all the carbohydrates and essential nutrients needed for the first four months. Of course, a baby on insulin will need regular carbohydrate to prevent hypos, so feeding little and often (around every three hours) during the day and four-hourly at night would be a typical timetable.

Mothers of small babies with diabetes naturally worry whether they can provide enough breast milk and this can become a vicious circle as anxiety can cause the milk flow to stop. Your diabetes specialist nurse will help you tackle this problem; you should be able to continue breast-feeding your baby but if he is not gaining enough weight, or has frequent hypos, you may need to supplement your breast milk with bottles between some breast feeds.

If the baby is growing very fast and is especially hungry you may need to introduce solids earlier than at the usual four months (this is often the case in babies without diabetes as well). In a baby with diabetes, solids will help slow down the absorption of milk sugar (lactose) which will be beneficial to blood glucose control.

Weaning a baby with diabetes onto solid food is no different from weaning any other baby. The baby should be given normal milk feeds with the kind of fruit or vegetable purées recommended for his age. Gluten-free foods (those without wheat) are recommended for all babies until they reach at least six months, when you can introduce him to a wider range of solid foods. It is now recommended that you do not introduce cow's milk until the baby is one year old. The BDA will supply you with a leaflet listing the food values of suitable baby foods, fresh or manufactured. All the popular shop-bought brands give a nutritional value chart on the packet or jar.

When the baby is one year old, a pattern should be established of three meals and two snacks in the daytime with an evening snack to cover the night-time insulin. As the baby will be drinking less milk now, the carbohydrate intake which previously came from milk will now come from the solid food.

It is well worth regular visits to your dietitian who will advise you on new tastes and suitable foods for the baby.

Weight Problems

Your baby's growth will be regularly checked at the hospital or clinic and recorded on height/weight charts. If the baby was underweight before diabetes was diagnosed, he will soon catch up. If a baby starts putting on too much weight then this will have to be discussed with the dietitian who may suggest cutting down on high-calorie fatty foods (see Chapter Six on Diet). Normally, though, a low-fat diet for children under five is not recommended.

Many babies are usually rather plump before they start walking, so don't worry too much until you can see that real exercise has started, at which time he should start losing that excess chubbiness.

Leading a Normal Life from the Start

Throughout this book we have talked about how important a normal lifestyle for the child with diabetes is, and babies are no different! The first few years of life will shape your child's view of the world. As every parent knows, it is only too easy to be over-protective. You may look at your baby and worry about the problems which you imagine lie ahead because of his diabetes and try to hold back his normal progress. That would be a big mistake. Don't discourage your child from learning to ride a bike, swim or play wild games with other children because you fear hypos. Your child should be encouraged to keep fit in every possible way, to try new experiences and get on with life. You must 'let go' and let him do everything that his brothers and sisters or friends are able to do.

Remember that controlling blood sugars at this time of life is bound to be difficult. Very young children grow fast and are completely unpredictable in their moods and behaviour from one day to the next.

'Simon reached the terrible twos and was very difficult for about a year,' said one mother. 'He threw the worst tantrums I'd ever heard which, quite surprisingly, never had anything to do with diabetes. The tantrums didn't come at injection or blood test time, he wasn't about to have a hypo . . . they were for completely irrational things, just like any other two year old. I noticed that controlling his diabetes was particularly hard during that time. It seemed that the stress of the tantrums sent the blood sugars up.'

The strain of bringing up a baby who has diabetes is especially great, yet parents learn to cope admirably. So will *you*, however remote that possibility might seem at first. Of course you will feel anxious and despairing at times. But by giving your baby the treatment he needs to stay healthy (however much you hate assaulting him with needles), the freedom to blossom into a confident personality, and the guidelines to tell right from wrong, you will be doing the best job any parent can hope to do.

Chapter 13

What Can We Hope for Our Children?

*'All I can think about is a cure for my child –
surely it must be around the corner . . .?'*

*'If they can land men on the moon you would think
scientists could find a cure for diabetes . . .'*

*'I feel optimistic – medical breakthroughs seem to happen
so fast these days that I live in real hope for the future . . .'*

What Does the Future Hold?

There are two main reasons to hope that, in time, new developments will make insulin injections a thing of the past. Firstly, one cannot have a holiday from insulin: there can never be a day off. In the second place, no matter how hard one tries to keep good diabetic control there is always the worry of long-term complications.

You may have heard about the development of insulin nasal sprays and wonder whether this could be the alternative to injections. While it seems possible that these might be available in the next few years, there are certain problems that are likely to mean nasal sprays could not be used as a total alternative to injections. The absorption and irritation of the sensitive mucous membrane in the nose are the main handicaps.

As parents of a child with diabetes who has her lifetime ahead your choice for her would almost certainly be total freedom from the injection regime.

The major areas of active research going on at present are all aimed at eventually freeing people with diabetes from insulin injections while producing totally normal blood sugar control. They are:

- insulin pumps which take over the function of the pancreas
- drugs which modify the process which causes diabetes in the first place
- pancreatic transplants, notably of the islet cells which produce insulin.

The Problem with Pumps

Insulin pumps (which we have mentioned briefly in Chapter Three) remain a research tool. There are still important problems which prevent their wide acceptance. Only a very small number of people actually use pumps to control their diabetes at the moment.

Pumps can be divided into two distinct types which are known as 'open-loop' and 'closed-loop'. The closed-loop pumps are intended to replace all the functions of the pancreatic beta cells (and have actually been called artificial pancreases). That is to say, they continuously measure the blood sugar concentrations, calculate on a minute-to-minute basis how much insulin the body needs, and then infuse the right amount.

The very first artificial pancreases, which were developed in the mid-1970s, were huge and required a trolley to carry them! They consisted of a pump which continuously withdrew small volumes of blood from a vein in one arm, another pump which injected insulin into the other arm, and a computer which decided how much insulin was necessary. Such machines were totally impractical except for very short periods of time. They were limited by the amount of blood which they took and the fact that the person was tethered to the trolley! Not only that, constant supervision was necessary as they were notorious for problems with blood clotting.

By the early 1980s, the impracticality of these machines led to the first open-loop devices. These were far less sophisticated gadgets, but had the advantage that they were portable and practical. There was no attempt to measure the blood glucose level: that was up to the person with diabetes. Nor was there a computer to say how much insulin you needed: you had to use your brain for that. They consisted simply of a small battery-operated syringe pump (the size of a Walkman which clipped onto a belt) connected by a long thin plastic tube to a small needle which was pushed through the skin on the tummy and left in place for two to three days at a time.

The pumps took only quick-acting insulin. They had two settings, a 'basal' rate at which there was a steady slow trickle of insulin, and a 'bolus' setting which you pressed before you ate. This infused insulin at a much faster rate, but for only a short period of time. The whole effect on circulating insulin concentrations was very similar to that found with an insulin pen. If anything, the results were slightly better overnight, when the constant rate of infusion prevented any problems with the insulin 'peaking' in the small hours, or wearing off before morning.

Extremely good control *is* possible with such pumps, but there is a price to be paid. Far from taking over the 'decision' of insulin doses these pumps actually make matters worse. You have to constantly do finger-prick blood tests and worry how much insulin to tell the pump to put in. Also, there is no reservoir of long-acting insulin under the skin, so if for any reason the insulin infusion is interrupted, blood glucose control gets worse very rapidly and there is a risk of ketosis.

To manage well with such pumps necessitated a fairly obsessional personality! They are also expensive. Insulin pens have largely superseded them since they are far more practical and can give control which is virtually as good. A major trial is currently under way in the United States comparing pumps with pens (using conventional insulin therapy) and looking at the risk of long-term diabetic complications. If it turns out that pumps can provide such really tight control as to make a great difference in the long term, we may yet see them make a comeback.

The ultimate goal, however, is a small portable closed-loop pump. This would require a miniature glucose sensor to give a constant readout of blood glucose levels. Such a pump was developed by the Jápanese as long ago as 1984. It used a sensor which was implanted under the skin, but this unfortunately became coated with the body's natural protein after only a few days. The Japanese do not yet seem to have found a way round this technical hitch and attempts are now being made to develop sensors which read the blood sugar level through the skin, via a beam of infra-red light.

Drug Possibilities

It used to be thought that the onset of diabetes was sudden: and indeed it is in terms of the symptoms. But although children who develop diabetes have rarely shown their symptoms for more than a few weeks, it is now recognised that in many cases it is possible to identify abnormalities many months or even years before the diabetes actually declares itself. The existence of this so-called *prodromal phase* raises the theory that it may be possible to interfere with the underlying process of destruction and prevent progression to actual diabetes.

In diabetes, the destruction of the beta cells in the pancreas is limited: no other organ is involved. Indeed, even the rest of the pancreas is unaffected. It is an immune disease caused by special cells, called T cells, whose function is to protect the body from foreign substances. The cells are involved, for example, in the rejection of grafts or transplants, and in diabetes it is just as if the T cells had been told that the child's own pancreas was a foreign body. This results in the formation of antibodies to the beta cells, and ultimately, to their destruction.

Several drugs are available which suppress or modify this immune process. These are drugs which have been developed for use in the treatment of patients who have had transplant operations, and they include steroids, azathioprine and cyclosporin. Several trials have shown that, alone or in combination, they are capable of exerting a major effect on the course of diabetes. Why then are these drugs not used much more widely?

The first difficulty, of course, is in identifying children who are going to develop diabetes. If there were some simple genetic marker which identified children at risk it would be one thing. But it is increasingly being recognised that genetic (or hereditary) factors play less of a role than had previously been thought, so that even if you have an identical twin with diabetes, *your* chances of developing the disease are not great. Furthermore, diabetes has a striking geographical distribution (increasing in the Northern Hemisphere) and a seasonal incidence, further suggesting the importance of environmental factors.

What happens if you wait until the diabetes develops and then treat the child immediately with drugs? At that stage, although there has already been a lot of damage to the beta cells (and the remaining cells look pretty sick) they are, in theory, capable of recovery if one could 'turn-off' the T cells. The interpretation of studies which have investigated this is not helped by the fact that insulin alone improves the functioning of the beta cells, so that after three months of insulin therapy up to 25% of children experience the 'honeymoon phase' and are able to discontinue insulin briefly, while many more have greatly reduced insulin requirements.

This honeymoon phase is exaggerated if children are also given the drug cyclosporin, so that 35% of children are able to come off insulin and the honeymoon phase is more prolonged, provided children are treated within the first few weeks of diagnosis. Unfortunately, however, there are problems; even in children who respond, the advantages are lost within a few weeks if the drug is stopped, implying that indefinite treatment would be needed. But the drug has side effects, some of which are cosmetic – like increased hair growth – but some of which are more serious, like the risk of damage to the kidneys and, ironically, the pancreas. On top of that, unless you are one of the lucky ones who can discontinue insulin completely, cyclosporin does not help much: if you are going to need insulin at all, there is no real advantage in needing a smaller dose.

The other drugs are even more toxic. Azathioprine affects the bone marrow and the liver, while steroids affect growth, cause weight gain and bone problems. They also irritate the effects of insulin, and make the person with diabetes prone to infections.

Basically, the price which has to be paid to put off the onset of diabetes is, at this moment in time, too high. We have not yet reached the point where we have the ability to turn diabetes around easily, and it will be only by careful research studies that these approaches can be extended. Yet the studies which have been done so far suggest that the underlying approach may be correct. Hopefully the development of more specific drugs, with fewer side effects, will make such an approach a practical possibility within a few years, particularly if we also get better at identifying the children at risk before they have symptoms of diabetes.

Different Types of Transplants

Diabetes results from failure of the beta cells of the pancreas. Why not simply replace them? After all, kidney transplants are done in patients whose kidneys have failed, and heart and liver transplants, while not as common, are also now quite possible.

The first pancreatic transplant was done in 1966, and early results with the technique were not good. This was mainly because you have to transplant the whole pancreas, most of which consists of a gland which secretes digestive enzymes. So long as these enzymes are secreted into the gut, where they perform their natural function of digesting food, all is well. But as soon as you handle the pancreas, temporarily deprive it of its blood supply and insert it into a foreign environment, it has a tendency to release its enzymes into the surrounding tissues, digesting anything within reach.

A major advance came in the late 1970s with the discovery of ways of blocking the tube carrying the digestive juices. This kills the cells which secrete enzymes, so that although the whole pancreas is transplanted, only the islets survive. Well over 1000 transplants have now been done, and when the technique works the diabetes is cured: the patient no longer needs insulin and his blood sugar levels are entirely normal. Yet the role of pancreatic transplantation is still far from certain.

Firstly, even now, only some 50% of grafts are still working one year after the operation. These results are not nearly as good as those obtained routinely with kidney transplants. In some cases, failure appears to be due to a recurrence of the process which caused the diabetes in the first place. Secondly, it is far from clear exactly *who* should be offered a pancreatic transplant. As with so many new procedures, the operation has tended to be done in patients who have had other medical problems and whose outlook is therefore not very good, and this may partly be why the results of pancreatic transplantation have not been better. One thing which is clear, though, is that existing diabetic complications are not reversed, after the transplant, despite impeccable diabetic control. Thirdly, following transplantation, patients require long-term treatment with the immuno-suppressive drugs which we have talked about earlier and, although the introduction of cyclosporin has greatly reduced the risk of side effects, these drugs are by no means benign. No formal trial has yet been done to compare the risks and benefits of pancreatic transplantation.

A recent alternative to transplantation of the whole pancreas is the transplantation of isolated islets, and much research is currently being done on this. The pancreas to be transplanted is deliberately digested with an enzyme solution, the islets are isolated and purified, and can then be injected as a 'soup'. This means that the necessary surgery is of a far more minor nature and raises the possibility of performing the transplantation much earlier in the disease – right at the beginning would be ideal.

It is very difficult to get the islets sufficiently pure, and many are lost in the process. This means that the number of islets which can be obtained from a pancreas is relatively small, and in humans the numbers of islets transplanted have been insufficient. Consequently the results have so far been a little disappointing. Very few patients have been able to come off insulin, and none have yet succeeded in achieving long-term survival of islet transplants comparable with whole pancreas transplants.

Yet there are some grounds for optimism. Firstly, the isolation of the islets in the test tube before transplantation makes some tricks possible. For example, attempts are being made to modify the islets before transplantation to make them better tolerated by the patient. Secondly, attempts are being made to use foetal islets. Obviously this raises moral issues, but foetal islets can be made to multiply in culture (and probably also in the body after transplantation) so that many more islets can be implanted. A recent publication from China has claimed that out of three hundred patients with diabetes given foetal islet transplants, twelve have been able to stop their insulin.

Conclusion

All of the techniques discussed above have been in development for over ten years, yet all still have major drawbacks. No-one should expect a sudden, dramatic cure for diabetes within the immediate future. Yet each year there are significant advances in our understanding of what causes diabetes, in our ability to prevent rejection of transplants and in the biotechnology necessary for artificial pancreases. Although research progress can at times seem painfully slow, it seems likely that developments in one or more of these areas will occur in the not-too-distant future which will make a major difference to the way we treat diabetes.

The future for your child with diabetes has never looked more exciting!

USEFUL ADDRESSES

Below are some useful contacts for you and your child. Several of the companies mentioned supply special literature for children to read and 'goodies' such as stickers and colouring books for them to enjoy. They can also keep you up to date on their latest available equipment.

Bayer Diagnostics UK   Tel: 0256 29181
Evans House
Hamilton Close
Basingstoke
Hants RG21 2YE
The Ames division manufacture blood sugar testing equipment and cater for children with all sorts of literature featuring Rupert Bear, comics and stickers.

Becton Dickinson   Tel: 0865 777722
Between Towns Road
Cowley
Oxford OX4 3LY
Manufacturers of needles and disposable syringes. Although these are mostly available on prescription, B-D can supply the thirty-unit syringes mentioned in Chapter Three which, at the time of writing, are not available on prescription. They are specially designed for children's small hands.

Boehringer Mannheim UK   Tel: 0273 480444
Bell lane
Lewes
East Sussex BN7 1LG
Manufacturers of blood sugar testing equipment. They supply literature for children and even do a boxed kit of blood testing meter and trendy bumbag.

British Diabetic Association (BDA)   Tel: 071 323 1531
10 Queen Anne Street
London W1M 0BD
National organisation providing links between diabetics and their families and publishing latest information on care and treatment.

Hypoguard (UK) Ltd   Tel: 03943 87333/4
Dock Lane
Melton
Woodbridge
Suffolk IP12 1PE
Supplies blood sugar testing equipment.

Medic-Alert Foundation   Tel: 071 833 3034
12 Bridge Wharf
156 Caledonian Road
London N1 9RD
Supplies identification bracelets and necklaces with conditions engraved on them.

MediSense Britain Ltd   Tel: 0675 467044
17 The Courtyard
Gorsey Lane
Coles Hill
Birmingham B46 1JA
Makes Exactech blood sugar testing equipment including pen sensor
which particularly appeals to children.

Novo Nordisk Pharmaceuticals Ltd   Tel: 0293 613555
Novo Nordisk House
Broadfield Park
Brighton Road
Pease Pottage
Crawley
West Sussex RH11 9RT
Insulin manufacturing company which operates a special youth scheme
which teenagers can join. Also runs Superskills in conjunction with many
hospitals and clinics (contact them if yours does not). This is a special
series of questionnaires designed to encourage the child to learn as much
about diabetes as possible. There are four 'papers' and each correct section
is rewarded with a smart enamel star badge and certificate.

Owen Mumford Ltd   Tel: 0993 812021
(Medical Shop)
Brook Hill
Woodstock
Oxford OX7 1TU
Supplies blood sugar testing equipment and accessories. Contact them for
a brochure which includes all kinds of carrying equipment.

SOS/Talisman   Tel: 0795 663403
Golden Key Co Ltd
1 Hare Street
Sheerness
Kent ME12 1AH
Supplies identification jewellery with a special range designed for children
depicting their favourite sports.

BIBLIOGRAPHY

Department of Health and Social Security, Report 28: *Diet in Relation to
Cardiovascular Disease*, 1984.
'Dietary Recommendations for Children and Adolescents with Diabetes',
British Diabetic Association, reprinted from *Diabetic Medicine*, journal of
the British Diabetic Association, 1989.
Various British Diabetic Association information and literature.

INDEX

Index